GETTING PREGNANT

Robert Winston is Director of the Infertility Clinic at Hammersmith Hospital, London, the largest comprehensive infertility clinic in Europe. He has written numerous specialist papers on infertility and holds the prestigious post of Professor of Fertility Studies at the University of London. Professor Winston is married with three children. He was presenter of the award-winning television series *Your Life In Their Hands* and is a regular contributor to radio and television programmes.

ROBERT WINSTON

Getting Pregnant

THE GUIDE TO INFERTILITY

PAN BOOKS

First published 1989 by Anaya Publishers Limited

This revised edition published 1993 by Pan Books
an imprint of Pan Macmillan Ltd
Pan Macmillan, 20 New Wharf Road, London N1 9RR
Basingstoke and Oxford
Associated companies throughout the world
www.panmacmillan.com

ISBN 0 330 32766 6

Text copyright © Robert Winston, 1989, 1993
Illustrations copyright © Lucy Su 1993

13 15 17 19 18 16 14

A CIP catalogue record for this book is available from
the British Library.

Typeset by Cambridge Composing (UK) Limited, Cambridge
Printed and bound in Great Britain by
Mackays of Chatham PLC, Chatham, Kent

This edition is dedicated to my friend, Donatella Flick, whose warmth, extraordinary generosity and kindness has made so much of our work at Hammersmith Hospital possible. By their support and encouragement, she and Muck Flick have greatly benefited our patients, and their friendship and understanding has meant a very great deal to me.

CONTENTS

PREFACE TO THIS EDITION

In the first edition of this book, I tended to shun technical language, preferring 'womb' for uterus, for example. This now seems really unnecessary and patronising. I therefore have reverted to common medical terms where they are in general usage. I have tried where possible to speak directly to the reader. In this earlier edition, I frequently wrote in the second person 'you'. On re-reading this, this approach now seems gauche. When I am trying to offer advice to infertile couples, some parts of this book specifically address men, at other times women, but mostly both. I hope that the change of emphasis does not depersonalise my approach. In the section on miscarriage, I still frequently refer to 'you', because this is an intense, personal experience and, to some extent, it is that aspect I am trying to explore.

Much of the book has been heavily rewritten; some of the more medical aspects have been pared down and the ethical, historical and research aspects have been considerably expanded, because most readers seem to find them interesting and, on occasions, amusing. My apologies if some of the stories alarm or disgust; my old chiefs were like this; often really larger than life.

I am indebted to the many members of my team, not least because they, like me, see the funny side of our work together. I am grateful to Kate Hardy and to Joe Conaghan, two of our scientists, with whom I enjoyed bouncing some of these ideas around. I must thank Raul Margara and other team members who got on with the work whilst I was occupied.

Finally, I want to express my love and gratitude to my wife Lira and children, Tanya, Joel and Benjamin, who tolerate my locking myself away with great generosity, during my various episodes of writing.

INTRODUCTION

How we have children is the most remarkable and, in many ways, mysterious of all our bodily functions. The desire to have children runs deeper than many of us realise or will admit. Whether one is religious or not, it is striking that the first command in the Bible is: 'Be fruitful and multiply' (Genesis 1: 28). Why we feel so strongly is not easy to explain.

One thing is clear. By having children, we leave a part of ourselves – our own genetic message which we inherited from our parents and they from their parents – on this planet. Our children are our connection with life that preceded us and that which follows us. It is truly remarkable that the unique collection of genes that we each have, which determine the way we think, the personality we have, the way we look, our abilities and disabilities, are identical to the genes carried right back to Abraham of the Chaldees, indeed to the very beginning of human existence. The processes involved in reproduction ensure that the genes of our parents are mixed and randomly assigned to us. These genes are reallocated in successive generations. Nature reshuffles the genetic pack with each conception.

Whatever we achieve on this Earth – even if, for example, we are politicians or Nobel Prize winners – becomes insignificant within fifteen years of our death. Try to name six Nobel Prize winners or six leading members of the government of fifteen to twenty years ago to see how quickly we forget what they achieved. But no matter how important or insignificant each of us is, we shape and contribute to the world of the future by producing a child.

How pregnancy occurs is remarkably complex and well over half the biological facts are still unknown. Much more research is required before we will know most of what there is to know about getting pregnant. This, above all, is why the treatment of people who have difficulty conceiving a child is so imperfect. I have written this book to try to explain how conception occurs because I find it riveting. For those having difficulty in conceiving, this book may also help maximise the chances of being fortunate. Whatever your motives, I hope you also find this subject as exciting, poignant and entertaining as I do because its implications are crucial for all human society.

PART ONE

BECOMING PREGNANT

CHAPTER ONE

How a Baby is Conceived

According to statistics recently published by the World Health Organization (WHO), over 100 million acts of sexual intercourse[1] take place each day. These result in around 910,000 conceptions, of which approximately 50 per cent are unplanned and 25 per cent definitely unwanted. About 150,000 unwanted pregnancies are terminated every day in the world, often in extremely unsafe conditions, and this results in approximately 500 deaths daily. 1,370 women die daily actually giving birth, some 25,000 infants and 14,000 children aged between one and four years die each day – 1 in 12 babies born this year will not see their first birthday. Sexually transmitted diseases are a serious problem worldwide: it is calculated that there are at least 130 million new cases each year of serious infection, and it is thought that there may currently be as many as 12 million cases of human immunodeficiency virus (HIV), leading eventually to AIDS which as far as we know is invariably fatal. Between 2 and 10 per cent of couples are unable to conceive any living child, and a further 10–25 per cent are unable to have a second or subsequent child. About one-third of all these cases is due to a problem with the man, and possibly another third due entirely to a problem only in the woman. WHO believes that somewhere between 60 and 80 million couples in the world are infertile.

These dry figures should make grim reading, for at the very

[1] WHO does not inform us as to whether the Earth actually moves as a consequence.

least, reproductive problems so frequently cause great unhappiness or deep suffering. Against this background there is remarkable ignorance about how humans conceive or what may go wrong. We are lucky, because most of us live in a society which has shielded us from the worst aspects of reproductive disease. Moreover, great advances are being made in human fertility problems, which should be of great benefit to us as individuals, and also to society as a whole. None the less, there is still great ignorance, prejudice and mystery about how we get pregnant; without accurate knowledge we remain powerless to change things for the better.

A good way to start learning about conception and how it occurs is to understand the more scientific aspects of human reproduction – how sperm meets egg and how the early embryo implants. Knowledge of this basic biology is fairly essential if we are to make sensible decisions about conception and contraception, and how to maximise the chances of normal development of an early pregnancy. What may come as a surprise is just how big are the gaps in what is known about getting pregnant.

I have tried three approaches in this chapter. First, I have devoted most space to those parts of human biology which are important medically. For example, to understand what the Fallopian tubes do may seem very unimportant. However, if you are unfortunate in having blocked or damaged tubes, it may help to know what functions and events should be taking place normally.

Second, I have, here and elsewhere, deliberately spent some time discussing animals other than humans. Apart from being interesting in itself, much of the knowledge we have about our own bodies comes from intensive studies of many animal species. Without those, we would be quite unable to make deductions about human physiology or understand how the human body works.

Third, whenever possible I have taken a look at the historical context. The history of our knowledge of human reproduction is extraordinary, fascinating and revealing. It tells us, apart from anything else, that we still suffer from many mistaken ideas even now, in an age of supposed enlightenment and sophistication.

The female reproductive system

THE EGGS

William Harvey's famous treatise *De generatione animalium (On the reproduction of animals)*, published in 1651, has a delightful frontispiece.

The hands of Jove hold an open egg, out of which come forth all forms of life. The egg, which perhaps is the beginning of all life, is as good a point as any for us to start.

Eggs (ova) do not simply grow in a woman's ovaries throughout her reproductive lifetime. The process which produces them begins when the human female embryo is less than 2 millimetres in length only about twenty-one days after fertilisation. Two millimetres is about half the size of the head of a match. It may seem slightly incredible that anything that small can have an egg in it, but human eggs are very small indeed, about one-tenth of the size of the full stop at the end of this sentence. Nevertheless, they are the largest cells in the human body.

At this stage of development, the female embryo has no clearly identifiable organs, although a primitive heart of some kind could be seen under a microscope. The cells from which the eggs will actually develop are called the *primordial germ cells*. These do not come from the embryo itself, but grow in the structure which in humans is next to the embryo – the *yolk sac*. It is thought that, about three weeks or so after fertilisation, these germ cells form up in line and move into the embryo along the structure which later in pregnancy will become the umbilical cord.

This procession of the germ cells is poorly understood. Certainly it is very remarkable, for it seems that the germ cells

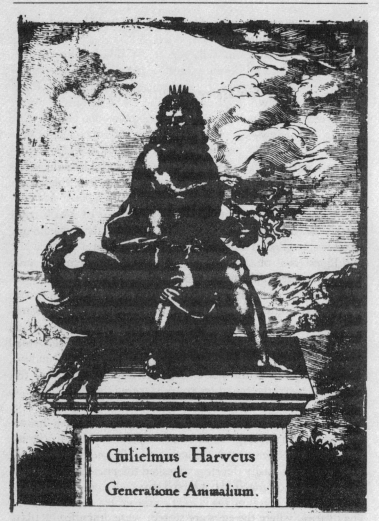

Gulielmus Harveus
de
Generatione Animalium.

Frontispiece from William Harvey's *On the reproduction of animals.*

move under their own steam towards the tissues which will
become the ovaries. In studies of animals, using time-lapse
photography, the germ cells have been seen to move rather like
an amoeba. As far as we know, only about 100 germ cells

migrate to the area which will become the ovaries, and there they continue to multiply.

The primordial germ cells repeatedly divide, and by the fifth month of life inside the womb, a baby girl has around 7 million eggs in her ovaries. By the time she is born, more than half of these eggs will have died and there will be only about 3 million left, and by puberty, only 400,000–500,000 remain. Of all these, only a few – no more than 400 or 500 (one each month or so) – will actually be ovulated during adult life. During a woman's fertile years – with time off for childbearing and breastfeeding – the maximum number of children she could have is only about thirty. According to the *Guinness Book of Records*, the world record is currently held by Mrs McNaught with twenty-two babies from twenty-two separate pregnancies. However, in the average adult relationship in the Western world, just two or three eggs will be properly fertilised and become children. When one considers that each of an adult woman's eggs is entirely genetically unique, with different genes derived at random from the woman's mother and father, nature does seem extraordinarily wasteful.

By the time of ovulation, when the egg leaves the ovary perhaps on its way to be fertilised, it contains only half the normal forty-six chromosomes that all other adult cells have – namely twenty-three. The other twenty-three will be contributed by the sperm which fertilises it. These chromosomes carry many thousands of genes and they determine the genetic make-up of the baby, deciding its unique characteristics as it develops.

THE OVARIES

The ovaries, where the eggs are stored, were described in 1651 by that great English physician William Harvey, who was very interested in reproduction. He had often accompanied Charles I when the King hunted deer on the royal estates. After the deer were killed, Harvey had been able to dissect them. 'The female testicles as they are called,' he wrote, 'whether they be examined before or after intercourse, neither swell nor vary from their

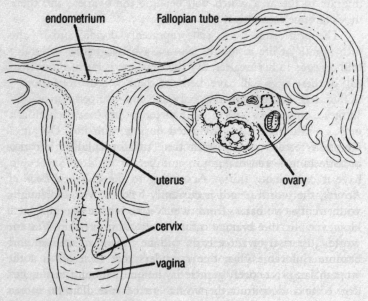

The female reproductive system.

usual condition; they show no trace of being of the slightest use either in the business of intercourse or in that of generation.' Fellows of the Royal Society, even to this day, get things wrong, and Harvey started a trend. His observations significantly held up progress in the understanding of reproduction. Today, we know much more, despite Harvey. For instance, we know that a girl's ovaries are hardly active at all during childhood. The length of time that the eggs remain in the ovaries in humans may be of particular significance. We know that both the primordial germ cells and the early eggs are very sensitive to certain physical stimuli such as radiation. The fact that, in humans, the eggs shed towards the end of reproductive life will have been in the ovary for forty years or longer may have some bearing on why older women are at greater risk of conceiving a genetically damaged child.

The ovaries remain immature and relatively inactive until puberty, when the pituitary gland – the 'master' of all the

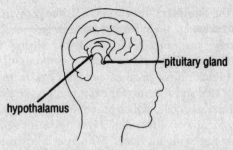

The pituitary gland and the hypothalamus in.the brain work together to produce hormones that regulate ovulation.

hormone-producing endocrine glands – starts to send messages to them. The pituitary gland, which is about the size of a small bean, is under the brain about an inch (2.5 cm) behind the eye sockets. Precisely what tells the pituitary gland to start sending hormone messages is not fully understood. It seems that the hypothalamus, a control centre in the brain about 3 inches (7.5 cm) behind the pituitary, plays a crucial role. The hormones which the pituitary produces are *follicle stimulating hormone* (FSH) and *luteinising hormone* (LH).

Follicle stimulating hormone is responsible for stimulating eggs to become mature. I pointed out earlier that there will be many thousands of eggs in each ovary. All of these inactive eggs are exposed to FSH from the pituitary at the time of puberty, but we do not understand why only a few of them start to respond to the stimulus to develop. Each egg which matures does so inside a small blister-like structure – the *Graafian follicle* – which is filled with fluid. The egg usually grows to one side of the follicle, where it is surrounded by helper cells – the *granulosa cells*.

Most eggs remain inactive and never develop inside an expanding follicle. Only those that do are capable of ovulation – that is, capable of leaving one of the ovaries and travelling through a Fallopian tube to be fertilised by a sperm. Each month, about twenty eggs, each within a follicle, start to mature, but in humans only one follicle becomes 'dominant' and goes on to become fully mature and to ovulate. As far as we know, the dominant follicle controls the growth of the other follicles and prevents them from getting large enoush to ovulate. Consequently, the other follicles actually shrink and the egg inside them dies. Only a few other mammals make a single dominant follicle; most produce several eggs at one ovulation. This is why cats and rabbits, for example, produce litters.

The granulosa cells, which surround each egg and line each follicle, perform two functions. First, they are responsible for feeding the egg with nutrients. The egg is virtually a perfect sphere with quite a smooth surface, and therefore it has the smallest surface area possible for its size. Yet it is highly active and consumes a lot of energy, especially when finally maturing, just before ovulation. On the face of it, it might seem as if God didn't do a particularly good job in designing the egg because it has little to call on within its own structure to provide the energy it needs. However, the 7 million or more granulosa cells which are packed into each follicle are there partly to look after each egg. Their total surface area hugely increases the amount of energy which is available to the egg by absorption. This remarkable phenomenon must be the only example in the body of one virtually invisible cell being serviced by many millions of others.

The second major function of the granulosa cells is to manufacture oestrogen. Oestrogen is the female hormone which stimulates breast development, female body shape and fat, and the other female secondary sex characteristics. As we shall see later, the levels of oestrogen in the body rise and fall during the menstrual cycle, depending on the number and activity of the granulosa cells.

OVULATION

Ovulation is when the egg leaves the ovary – in humans, roughly halfway between two menstrual periods. In all mammals this process is controlled by the hormones from the pituitary gland: LH and FSH. As we have seen, FSH stimulates the follicle to grow to its maximum, before ovulation. LH then

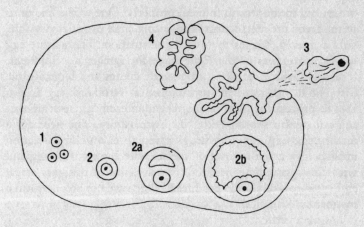

The development of a follicle containing the egg. (1) Immature eggs. (2, 2a & 2b) Maturing Graafian follicle and egg. (3) Rupture of follicle with release of egg surrounded by granulosa cells (ovulation). (4) *Corpus luteum* about 4–5 days after ovulation.

stimulates the follicle to open and release the egg. How does the body know when to send the LH signal? There is a wonderful mechanism here. Understanding this helps us to understand what sometimes goes wrong when women fail to ovulate.

As FSH stimulates the follicle to grow, the granulosa cells (which produce oestrogen) increase in number and activity. As the granulosa cells increase, so does the manufacture of oestrogen. Eventually oestrogen output is high and causes a rise in the level in the bloodstream. This rise in oestrogen in the blood stimulates the brain, telling the hypothalamus that the follicle is now mature and ready to release a ripe egg. An immediate message is then sent from the hypothalamus to the pituitary gland. The pituitary responds by sending out a sharp pulse of LH, and approximately thirty-six hours after the rise of LH in the blood, ovulation occurs. This process – that is, the rise of one hormone promoting the secretion of another and so on – is called a 'feedback' mechanism.

Immature eggs will not normally fertilise. If they do, fertilisation produces an abnormal embryo which cannot survive or implant in the womb (uterus) properly. One of the functions of the feedback mechanism is to ensure that, as far as possible, only a ripe egg leaves the ovary at ovulation. The mature egg has chromosomes at the right stage for further development. It also is capable of taking in a single sperm and blocking the entry of all other sperm surrounding it. A mature egg is also able to process the head of the sperm entering it, ensuring that egg and sperm subsequently fuse successfully. The need for a mature egg explains why drugs given to encourage ovulation must be given in the right sequence, with the right timing and with the appropriate hormone tests. Without this, abnormal embryos are likely to be produced, which are not able to form a pregnancy.

THE EGG AFTER OVULATION

Once the egg has left its follicle, it hopefully will find its way into one of the Fallopian tubes. The end of each tube lies close to the surface of one of the ovaries. Whether the tube actively picks up the egg is unknown. It probably does, as the lining of the tube has very fine hair-like structures – *cilia* – which beat rhythmically, wafting any nearby particles into the tube itself. These cilia seem to be important as they undoubtedly provide one way in which eggs are transported down the tube and eventually into the uterus. When the cilia are damaged or missing – for example, after a tubal infection – a woman may be infertile or prone to ectopic pregnancy (*see* Chapter 13).

The egg has other assistance in its journey to meet the sperm. The egg is still surrounded by granulosa cells from the ovary, immediately after ovulation. These cells, which viewed under a microscope resemble a sunburst, probably help the egg find its way into the tube. They are very sticky and adhere to the tubal surface. Once the egg is in the tube, it is ready to meet the sperm.

People frequently wonder what happens if the egg does not, or cannot, find its way into the tube. This may be the situation, for example, if the tubes are blocked. In practice, it is very likely that eggs are frequently lost outside the tube. Even though they are the biggest, single cells in the body, they are still very tiny – invisible to the naked eye – and they simply get lost within the abdomen, where they disintegrate.

Let us now leave the egg, hopefully in the Fallopian tube, and return to the ovary.

THE OVARY AFTER OVULATION

Following ovulation, the follicle from which the egg came tends to fill with blood. This is one of the reasons why women sometimes feel some pain at the time of ovulation, although, to be fair, this pain can occasionally occur before ovulation with mere enlargement of the follicle. Indeed, this pain is no guarantee that ovulation has definitely occurred. The blood in the follicle forms a clot and is replaced with fibre-like tissue. The remaining granulosa cells, in addition to producing oestrogen, now start to produce a second hormone, *progesterone*. The production of progesterone is stimulated by the release of LH from the pituitary gland which occurred immediately before ovulation. As we shall see later, progesterone is the hormone which prepares the uterus for implantation of the developing embryo, if fertilisation occurs successfully.

The granulosa cells also make an orange-yellow pigment. This is quite vivid in colour, and it stains the entire ruptured follicle. The resulting structure is called a *corpus luteum* (literally 'yellow body' in Latin). This yellow appearance was first noted in 1562 by the great Italian anatomist Gabriel Fallopius[2] (who was the first to describe the tubes that were then named after him), but it wasn't until 1697 that the name *corpus luteum* was

[2] Canon of Modena Cathedral, before studying medicine in Ferrara, and thence to Pisa. He died, aged thirty-nine, in 1562 having made a number of important anatomical discoveries. For some reason he concentrated on the female genitalia and was responsible for naming the vagina and the clitoris. He was a vigorous critic of Galen (Greek second-century physician) whose dissections of the pig and Barbary ape – together with the Church's interdiction on human dissection – held up developments in human medicine for over 1,200 years, as Galen's observations were regarded as infallible.

coined, by another famous anatomist, Marcello Malpighi,[3] after he had described its detailed appearance in the cow. Its function has only recently been understood, and today research still goes on about precisely what it does. The *corpus luteum* is certainly a most important structure, as not only does it produce the progesterone needed to prepare the uterus for a possible pregnancy, but its progesterone production is essential for the earliest development of any embryo which forms. If the *corpus luteum* is damaged, an early pregnancy may miscarry.

MENSTRUATION

Why is it that human females menstruate, unlike the so-called 'lower' animals? All female mammals need to prepare the uterus so that a pregnancy will implant. In lower animals there is an *oestrus cycle* where the female comes on to heat and is receptive to the male. During this phase, which may be very frequent or very infrequent – once every four days in guinea pigs,[4] once a year in hippopotamuses – the lining of the uterus is prepared for the possible reception of a pregnancy.

In the evolution of humans and certain others of the monkey family, the oestrus cycle has been replaced by the menstrual cycle. Perhaps because, in humans, sexual intercourse is usually

[3] Marcello Malpighi (1628–1694), another of the great Italian scientists who founded the science of microscopy, examining many body tissues in extraordinary detail. One of his most important discoveries was the identification of the blood supply in the lungs. He was forced from Bologna because of envy and jealousy from his colleagues, and his remarkable studies continued to produce resentment in Sicily, where he then did research. His historic work on the chick embryo (1673) is of great importance, and in some respects his conclusions were similar to those of William Harvey. Ten years before his death, his house, books, manuscripts and microscope were all destroyed, and it was only at the end of his life that he was reinstated by Pope Innocent XII.

[4] Some scientists from Chile, who were nuns working at the Catholic University of Santiago, visited my laboratory because we were all interested in our various experiments on guinea pigs, and they wished to compare notes. We commiserated with each other, because it is difficult to tell when a guinea pig is ovulating; the sign is merely a slight, temporary opening of the vagina. When I observed that my guinea pigs open their vagina every four days, my visitors replied (in broken English), 'Why, ours open every three days.'

much more of a cerebral process (and not just a question of rutting), women do not simply become physically receptive to men as females of other species do to males. In humans, the female has far more control. It is the development of this degree of control which seems to have led to the evolution of the menstrual cycle.

Until the eighteenth century it was often supposed that women usually ovulated at the time of menstruation. This idea was based on the evidence that women who did not menstruate were usually infertile. It was also recognised that animals, who went through an oestrus period, ovulated at this time.

A clue to the truth was found in the post-mortem room. Although it was generally agreed that ovulation occurred during menstruation, doctors and scientists were puzzled because, during autopsies of women who had been menstruating at the time of their deaths, they could find little sign of any ovarian activity – and it was known that the egg developed in a follicle, a structure very obvious to the naked eye. On the other hand, follicles were sometimes seen at post-mortem in women who had not had a menstrual period for several years. In spite of these essentially conflicting pieces of evidence, doctors remained convinced that ovulation coincided with menstruation. Dr Pouchet, writing in Paris as late as 1842, stated that 'in the intermenstrual phase . . . conception is physically impossible.'

This led Dr Raciborski, also of Paris, to an ingenious idea. He interrogated a group of young women, all of whom had (presumably) been virgins before their marriages and who became pregnant within two months of their weddings. The majority of those marrying within a few days of the end of their period conceived immediately. Those who married 10–18 days after a period never conceived until the following month. Thus Dr Raciborski arrived successfully at the correct time of human ovulation. It says something for the stubborn nature of the medical profession that his observations were largely ignored. It is also interesting to think that, with the changes in sexual morality and the availability of contraception, his observations could not have been made in our present society.

WHY MENSTRUATION STOPS DURING PREGNANCY

The *corpus luteum* breaks down (degenerates) if it receives no stimulus. As LH production from the pituitary gland falls after ovulation, there is no longer any stimulus to the ovary, so the *corpus luteum* withers and progesterone production falls. The fall in progesterone leads to a loss of stimulus to the uterus, and its blood-filled lining therefore also withers. This produces menstrual bleeding. If a pregnancy occurs, the embryo produces the hormone *human chorionic gonadotrophin* (HCG). HCG is almost identical in chemical structure to LH, so similar, in fact, that the *corpus luteum* cannot tell the difference. Consequently, in the event of pregnancy, the *corpus luteum* is maintained, progesterone output carries on, the lining of the uterus continues to be stimulated and menstruation does not occur.

The male reproductive system

THE PRODUCTION OF SPERM

Unlike eggs, which are present in the ovaries from before birth, spermatozoa, or sperm, are first manufactured at puberty. They are made in the two tests (or testicles), the organs which hang inside the scrotum. The testes are filled with thousands of microscopic little tubes, inside which the sperm grow (*see* below). These minute tubes are connected to yet more tubes, called the *rete testis*. *Rete* is Latin for 'a net', and this term was given to this structure presumably because the fine tubes form a network in the testes. The tubes in the rete testis are thought to produce special fluids, important for sperm development. The rete in each testicle is connected to yet more tubes, called the *efferent ducts*, of which there are about eight. These efferent ducts lead into one single tube, the *epididymis*, which is itself a pretty amazing bit of plumbing.

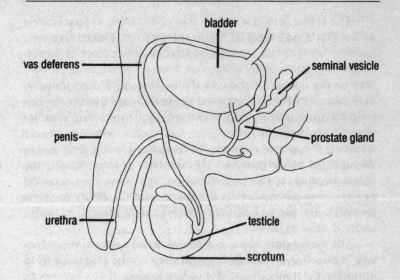

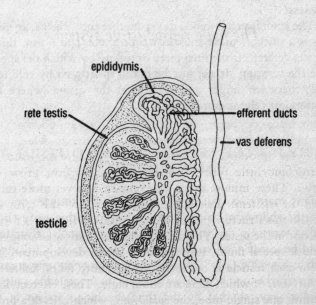

The male reproductive system.

The epididymis is a remarkably coiled tube, approximately 40 feet (12 m) in length. It has an extremely fine inner diameter, or bore, being thinner in total width than a fine piece of thread. Sperm are transported along this tubing, which is their only way to the outside world. At the beginning of their journey, they cannot move on their own; the epididymis itself is responsible for their transport by means of gentle muscular contractions in its wall. However, the epididymis does not simply transport the sperm; it also modifies them. During their travels through the epididymis, which take two to three weeks, the sperm become capable of fertilisation, and some ill-understood process takes place whereby the sperm gain the ability to move (*motility*). By the end of their journey, they are able to swim under their own power.

The epididymis, then, is a complex and essential reproductive organ. If it is damaged, sperm may not be able to develop normally and may be incapable of fertilisation. If blocked – even in only one tiny place – all sperm production from that testicle is useless.

The epididymis is joined to yet another tube, the *vas deferens*. This is a thicker, more muscular tube about 4 to 6 mm thick. The vas deferens is the final piece of tubing by which the sperm leave the scrotum. It can just be felt in most men by rolling it gently between finger and thumb in the groin, where the scrotum joins the abdominal skin.

WHY DO THE TESTICLES HANG OUTSIDE A MAN'S BODY?

In many mammals, but by no means all, the testicles descend from the abdominal cavity into a scrotum during early childhood. Once outside, they are considerably cooler than they would be inside. The temperature in the scrotum is usually as much as 8.5–15°F (4–7°C) below the general body temperature. Moreover, the blood vessels to the testicles are coiled in a highly complex way, so that by the time the blood arrives in the scrotum, it is much cooler than normal.

It is widely thought that the cooler temperature of the scrotum is essential for proper sperm production. It is this idea which leads to many men with poor sperm counts being asked to take regular cold baths. If you have been given this advice and you are reluctant to use cold water on this sensitive region, think of the bull elephant whose testicles are completely inside the abdomen, not I think, to the detriment of his power of procreation.

THE FINAL STAGE OF THE JOURNEY

Unlike the epididymis in the scrotum, the vas deferens moves the sperm along quite rapidly. It contracts during male orgasm and transports sperm past the *seminal vesicles* and the *prostate gland* into the urethra. The urethra is the tube which connects the bladder to the outside world, through the penis. During ejaculation, the opening between the urethra and the bladder shuts, and semen containing sperm is rapidly transported along it.

THE SEMEN

The semen is at first partly fluid, partly solid. It contains the sperm and a fluid component from the seminal vesicles and from the prostate gland. Some fluid is also contributed by glands in the urethra itself. All this fluid is essential to provide the sperm with energy. Men who have a damaged prostate or damaged seminal vesicles may be infertile. The solid component containing the sperm is in the form of a jelly and after ejaculation it remains in this form for up to thirty minutes. Liquefaction (the 'melting' of this jelly caused by a special chemical process) is necessary before the sperm are capable of release into the female genital tract.

EJACULATION

During orgasm, ejaculation follows a vigorous pumping action of the muscles at the base of the penis. In certain rare cases of infertility, these muscles may not work properly. The total volume of semen – the *ejaculate* – should usually be about 1–8 millilitres (an average teaspoon holds about 5 millilitres of fluid). If there is too little fluid, the man may be infertile because there is not enough fluid to carry the sperm into the female system; too much and the sperm may be too diluted. However, on the whole, the precise volume is usually not all that important, and is nothing for you and your partner to get worried about – certainly there is no need to raid the kitchen drawer for teaspoons to check the semen volume. Interestingly, most of the sperm are contained in the first part of ejaculation; the rest is just surplus fluid.

In some animals, such as rodents, the ejaculate remains solid for a considerable length of time, forming a jelly plug that fills the female's vagina. The quantity of fluid ejaculated varies considerably from species to species: in mice, only a minute droplet is ejaculated, while pigs may produce a cupful. The length of sexual intercourse also varies hugely: in bulls and rabbits it is over in a matter of seconds, while camels take twenty-four hours, which must be a source of great satisfaction in arid and featureless deserts.[5]

THE SPERM

Just as the egg is the largest cell in the body, the sperm are the smallest. They were first described in 1678 by Anthony Van Leeuwenhoek,[6] when he examined semen (possibly his own)

[5] The chap I feel sorry for is the male sphenodon, a rare, frightening-looking lizard from New Zealand and a close relative of the extinct dinosaurs. He is one of the only animals not to have a penis at all. Come to think of it, perhaps that's why dinosaurs died out.

[6] Dutch microscopist, 1632–1723. There is a fine portrait of him in the

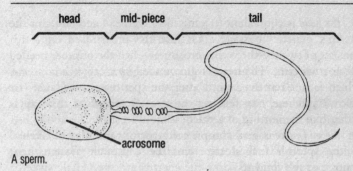

A sperm.

using a primitive microscope of his own design and making. Actually, as frequently happens in science, Van Leeuwenhoek, although credited with the discovery of human sperm, was not actually the first to see them. Nowadays it is largely forgotten that probably the first person to see sperm was Dr Louis Hamm in 1667, who had been using a microscope to study the nocturnal emissions of a patient with gonorrhoea. He then told Van Leeuwenhoek of his discovery of moving spermatozoa. The latter published a full description of his own findings, calling the sperm 'animalcules'. It rapidly became fashionable in well-to-do society for men to examine their own semen, and soon many people believed they could see a fully formed human figure (a *homunculus*) in the head of the sperm. Some people even wrote of having discovered male and female sperm under the microscope; others imagined they could see the sperm intertwined in microscopic intercourse or even pregnant.

It was only with the modern invention of the electron microscope that really detailed information about sperm was acquired. A sperm comprises three major parts and may be thought of as rather like a missile:

Rijksmuseum in Amsterdam. During his life he is said to have ground over 400 lenses, some of which were no larger than a pinhead; he is a faintly shadowy figure, and unlike Malpighi (*see* p. 16), kept his methods secret, presumably so that they could not be copied. He demonstrated his microscope to Queen Mary II of England, but whether he proudly showed her his sperm is not recorded.

● *the head* is equivalent to a missile's warhead and contains the sperm's genetic message. Just like the unfertilised egg, this consists of twenty-three chromosomes – half the number needed for normal cells. The head is surrounded by a cap, the *acrosome*, which is not removed until after the sperm is capacitated (*see* below) and ready to fertilise the egg. Removal of this cap is rather like the arming of a warhead;

● *the mid-piece* is very complex in structure and may be likened to the sperm's fuel storage and the computer systems that control its movements;

● *the tail*, which moves like a whiplash, provides the propulsive force which moves the sperm forward. The force of this whiplash increases greatly when the sperm is close to its target, the egg, when it accelerates considerably.

HOW EGG AND SPERM MEET

During sexual intercourse, the average man ejaculates between 100 million and 300 million sperm into the vagina. Quite remarkably, just as each human egg is unique, each of these sperm is genetically unique. Each contains a different set of genes, derived from those of the man, and, depending upon which sperm finally hits which egg, the resulting baby will exhibit its unique, individual characteristics.

This number of sperm may seem enormous, especially when it is realised that only one is required to fertilise an egg. Some species, such as pigs and cattle, actually produce far more – several thousand million at a single ejaculation. Many sperm are required because of the perilous journey they now undertake. How the egg and sperm finally meet is not simple. Some very recent evidence suggests that the egg may release chemicals which can be recognised by the sperm. The suggestion is that normal sperm may actually be attracted to the egg, almost as if they could 'smell' it.

To start with, many sperm simply fall out of the vagina. This is quite natural, but it can be of great concern to infertile couples who imagine that something abnormal is happening to them.[7]

Then, the vagina itself is relatively hostile to sperm. The vaginal secretions are rather acid, an environment in which sperm usually do not survive very easily. It may seem strange that nature has allowed the vagina to be acid, as reception of sperm is obviously crucial for the survival of the species. But this acidity also protects against bacteria and dangerous infection, and thus prevents damage to the lining of the uterus and tubes.

Some sperm – perhaps no more than 5 per cent – find their way into the mucus that covers the neck of the womb, or *cervix*. This mucus tends to be thin, watery and penetrable to sperm near the time of ovulation. Here, two important things happen to the sperm. First, they are protected, not only against the acids in the vagina, but also against the woman's white blood cells, including the *phagocytes*. These scavenging cells, which normally protect the body against invasion by bacteria and other foreign material, are not usually active in healthy cervical mucus around the time of ovulation. Second, during physical contact with the mucus, each sperm undergoes a quite mysterious process called *capacitation*, in which the sperm cap (the acrosome) is removed. Only when this has happened is the sperm capable of penetrating an egg. Within five to ten minutes of ejaculation, some sperm pass through the cervical mucus, through the uterus, and into the tubes, where they are ready to fertilise an egg. The remaining sperm in the cervical pool of mucus stay there for many hours – certainly seventy-two hours and possibly much longer – with sperm constantly being passed up into the uterus and then the tubes.

However, few sperm get into the uterus. Just how few is uncertain. We know that, in rabbits, perhaps not more than 0.5 per cent make it through the cervix. The situation is likely to be quite similar in women. Therefore, of the 300 million that

[7] It is this phenomenon which, I think, causes many couples to adopt different postures during intercourse. Some doctors recommend that the women lies with a pillow under her bottom, so that the semen is retained. There is no evidence at all that this improves the chance of conception.

arrived in the vagina, no more than 1–2 million at most get as far as the uterus.

The uterus is also a hostile environment. Here there are many phagocytes, protective against infection, which recognise the sperm as foreign invaders and thus set out to destroy them by swallowing most of them. Only a small fraction of sperm get into the Fallopian tube. At any one time, after intercourse, probably no more than about 200 sperm will be present.

Passage of sperm into the Fallopian tube seems a complicated affair. They do not swim there. They are actively transported, probably by muscular contractions of the uterus and tubes. We know this because the speed at which human sperm swim has been carefully measured. Considering the tiny size of the sperm, the distance from the cervix to the tube is huge and if sperm were left to their own travel arrangements, they would not arrive in the tube until seven or more hours after intercourse. In fact, sperm get into the tube within five minutes after being deposited in the vagina; this has been demonstrated in volunteers undergoing surgery on their Fallopian tubes. It is interesting to consider that, while the tube is transporting sperm in one direction – towards the ovary – it is simultaneously transporting the egg in precisely the opposite direction – towards the uterus and therefore the sperm pool. A complex tube, indeed.

As well as transporting sperm, the Fallopian tube also acts as a filter. The human male is an unusual animal in that he tends to produce many abnormal sperm in his ejaculate. The first part of the tube – the *isthmus* – appears to trap dead and abnormal sperm so that only normal ones arrive in the upper part – the *ampulla*.

Because sperm can live for quite long periods both in the cervical mucus and in the tubal fluids, careful timing of intercourse just before ovulation is almost certainly unnecessary. It is important to understand this, because recognition of this fact takes some of the sting out of being infertile. Many couples trying to conceive get very worried about timing intercourse. This can make sexual intercouse a far cry from love-making and creates a great strain for some people. Just how long the sperm are capable of fertilising an egg after intercourse is unknown –

perhaps two days or so. We know for certain that, in some species, sperm retain their viability for long periods. In some bats, for instance, sperm are definitely known to be retained in the uterus for several months after intercourse and are still able to cause a pregnancy. In a particular strain of mouse, the female can become pregnant with two successive litters after a single act of insemination. This is evidence that some of the sperm survive in the glands of the uterus throughout pregnancy before being finally allowed to fertilise eggs.

Fertilisation

FERTILISATION AND DEVELOPMENT OF THE EMBRYO

Fertilisation – the stages during which the sperm enters the egg and fuses with it and the egg starts dividing – takes place in the Fallopian tube. Fertilisation is not a single instantaneous process: in humans, it takes place over the best part of twenty-four hours. For entirely healthy fertilisation to occur, the egg has to be properly mature. If it is 'under-ripe', a sperm may not enter it properly; if 'over-ripe', more than one sperm may enter it, causing an abnormal number of chromosomes (i.e. more than forty-six), which is incompatible with life.

A mature egg has its chromosomes ready for cell division, and its chemistry ready to utilise the energy needed for subsequent cell division. A mature egg is also capable of only allowing a single sperm to penetrate it: remarkably, as soon as one sperm has penetrated, a normally mature egg throws up a chemical barrier which prevents other sperm from entering it. An abnormal or immature egg may divide into what may seem to be a normal embryo, but the embryo so formed will not go on to become a live baby. The factors which decide whether an egg is mature or not are largely hormonal; it is for this reason that measurement of a woman's hormones during 'test-tube baby' (in vitro fertilisation, IVF) treatment is so important.

Those IVF programmes in which blood hormone levels are not measured regularly (all too common, I'm afraid) may be unable to detect when the eggs that have been stimulated are properly mature (*see* Chapter 11).

The fertilised egg develops in the tube. During the first twenty-four hours it divides once into two cells. During the next day, each of those cells divides. Each cell division occurs at intervals of about fifteen hours so that, by the end of two days there are four to eight cells, and by the time ninety hours have elapsed there are usually somewhere around sixty-four cells. In the early stages of human development – that is, when the embryo comprises up to about eight cells – each cell has what is known as *totipotential*. This simply means that each cell contains all the capability of developing into a human being. Thus, if the eight-cell embryo was deliberately divided into its eight independent cells, which were then left to grow separately, potentially eight human beings – each, incidentally, identical – could develop. This is the mechanism by which identical twins occur; occasionally, the embryo divides completely into two, quite spontaneously.

The ability of each early embryonic cell to develop into a person is of considerable importance to women undergoing IVF treatment. Quite commonly, an embryo with several of its total number of cells fragmented or dying may be put deliberately into the uterus. Occasionally, seven cells out of a total of eight may show signs of not being viable. This does not necessarily prevent a perfectly normal pregnancy occurring, provided the one remaining cell is quite healthy. Another interesting fact is that an embryo, when it arrives in the uterus ninety-six hours or so after fertilisation, is composed of approximately 64–200 cells. Most of these cells, perhaps 85 per cent of them, become the membranes (in which the baby lives) and placenta (which nourishes it), and these are thrown away at birth! Only a very few cells, those comprising the so-called *inner cell mass*, actually develop into the embryo proper.

It is worth pointing out that an egg may divide into separate cells without ever having been exposed to a sperm. If this happens, the egg looks to all intents and purposes like a perfectly

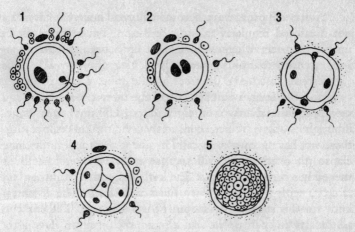

Fertilisation and early embryonic development. (1) Just one sperm enters the egg and others are immediately 'locked out'. The tail of the fertilising sperm breaks off. (2) Two pronuclei form about 15 hours after sperm entry and are only visible for a few hours. (3) The first division of the egg into two cells is completed in about 20–40 hours. (4) By 2–3 days the embryo may be approximately eight cells, each potentially capable of developing into a person. (5) By about 80 hours the blastocyst is formed, containing perhaps 50–100 cells.

normal embryo. This independent cell division, or *cleavage*, may be stimulated by exposure to electric shock, sudden changes in temperature or alteration in the chemical environment surrounding the egg; it can also occasionally happen without any obvious stimulus. Such cleaving eggs, at least in mammals, are not capable of development beyond a certain stage. For one thing, most of them will not have the correct numbr of chromosomes. However, in frogs, such a cleaved egg (which has never even seen a sperm) is capable of developing into a perfectly healthy adult frog – a true example of virgin birth. The technical term for this is 'parthenogenesis'. Spontaneous cleavage of eggs is important because an unfertilised but cleaved egg may be mistaken for a normal embryo and transferred to the uterus during test-tube baby treatment. Unless the egg is examined approximately eighteen hours after exposure to sperm, it is not possible to know until later whether an egg (which may appear to have become a normal embryo) has really been fertilised. For this reason, the best test-tube baby clinics always examine all eggs about eighteen hours after insemination, to ensure that only potentially viable embryos will later be transferred.

After the human embryo enters the uterus, it floats around for approximately two or three days. Up until this stage, although its cells have been constantly dividing and multiplying, it will not have grown physically in size at all. It is still the same size as the original egg cell because each cell which has been formed has been smaller than the last. It is now a clump or ball of cells, with a central cavity filled with fluid. The technical name for this stage of development is a *blastocyst*. The embryo only starts to increase in size around six or seven days after fertilisation, just about the time when it starts to stick to the lining of the uterus, the *endometrium*.

Not all mammals follow the same pattern as humans. In some species, the free-floating embryo at the blastocyst stage goes into a kind of suspended animation – so-called 'diapause'. This period of suspension of all growth or activity varies considerably from species to species: in roe deer, the embryo almost stops all development for five months and pregnancy lasts for a total of about ten months. In European badgers, the embryo halts all growth at this stage for ten months, being simply retained in the mother's uterus. The longest example of suspended animation is in the wallaby, a member of the kangaroo family, where embryonic growth is halted for up to a year. Why diapause should occur in some species is not entirely known, but it is widely believed that this is an adaption to a harsh environment, and prevents young being born during the depths of a bitter winter, when their chances of survival would be seriously limited.

IMPLANTATION OF THE EMBRYO

Seven days after fertilisation, the human embryo starts to implant into the endometrium. Precisely how this happens is not

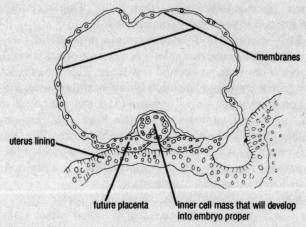

membranes

uterus lining

future placenta   inner cell mass that will develop
into embryo proper

The start of implantation of a 7-day embryo into the lining of the uterus, here seen in cross-section. Most of the embryonic cells form the placenta and membranes, and only about one-tenth will become a person (if implantation succeeds).

at all well understood at present. It is a major area of research, one that has the most important implications in our understanding of normal fertility, infertility, miscarriage and contraception, and one in which we can, hopefully, expect greater progress during the next decade. The embryo appears to control its own implantation and, apparently, it does this by secreting the pregnancy hormone human chorionic gonadotrophin (HCG). As we have already seen, this is the hormone which is very similar in structure to the pituitary hormone LH, which stimulates the ovary to make progesterone.

HCG appears to influence the lining of the uterus to receive the embryo and allow it to implant. HCG can be detected soon after this stage by very sensitive pregnancy tests on blood – even before the next menstrual period is due. Implantation is a very remarkable event. The embryo is completely foreign. It is going to become an individual quite different from its mother, with its own blood group, tissue type and special proteins. However, it is not rejected by the mother's body. It is, in fact, the perfect transplant – the perfect parasite. No other foreign material is ever accepted as readily, because the body's natural defence mechanisms will prevent it. This extraordinary phenomenon is very poorly understood.

Early embryonic development and implantation are very precarious. We know that at least 40 per cent of human embryos simply do not make it beyond this stage. This information has been gained by doing sensitive blood hormone tests for very early pregnancy just before menstruation in a number of volunteers. Surprising numbers of women have a weakly positive test, but they bleed normally shortly afterwards. Why they do this is not clear. It seems that many embryos are lost at the time of menstruation, just as early implantation is completed; this phenomenon is not really understood.

A slightly delayed, heavier-than-usual period signifies that a very early pregnancy has been lost. Women who occasionally experience delayed cycles when they think they have definitely ovulated, may well be getting pregnant but losing the early embryo. It is well worth finding out, therefore, if conception is actually happening. A sensitive blood test for HCG may be greatly reassuring because it shows that one is at least capable of getting pregnant – especially after tubal surgery, for example, when this knowledge will give real and genuine hope.

By fourteen days, the tiny embryo is firmly implanted in the uterine lining. Although miscarriage can still happen, it is now much less likely, and it becomes progressively less common the further a pregnancy develops (see Chapter 13). It is at this point that the organs of the embryo first start to develop. The 'primitive streak', the beginning of the nervous system, is the first identifiable structure. The heart starts to form at around twenty-three days and other organs follow. The baby has a clearly defined human shape by about ten weeks, when it is almost 1 inch (2.5 cm) long and weighs about ¼ ounce (7 g).

CHAPTER TWO

Timing a Pregnancy

Most people simply do not consciously plan a pregnancy and families are no worse off for that. As we have seen the statistical chance of getting pregnant in any given month is really surprisingly low. The vagaries of our biology and the fact that humans are the most naturally infertile of all mammals makes the achievement of a pregnancy an imprecise and unpredictable event. This has led to a wealth of mythology about human conception.

Students of archaeology and architecture may be aware of the fine historic buildings of County Durham. Nikolaus Pevsner has written of Finchale Priory, a monastery established for eight monks and an abbot in AD 1196. This was modernised in 1460 when the famous Douglas Tower was built. Here there is an oriel window, under which there was built a stone seat. A piece of rude folklore (according to Pevsner) surrounds this seat which was said to have the virtue of removing sterility and procuring issue for any woman who, 'having performed certain ceremonies, sat down thereon'. Regrettably, Henry VIII dissolved the English monasteries and got rid of all the monks in 1533. Oddly, since that date the seat has been observed to have entirely lost its efficacy.

A much more recent example of pregnancy timing, also from the north of England, has recently come to my attention. The much respected *Today* programme (BBC Radio 4) recently reported on the Asda supermarket in Widnes, Lancashire. Apparently, interesting phenomena have surrounded check-out till number 15. In the last twenty-two years, no fewer than thirty-three check-out girls on that till have got pregnant. Indeed, some of the shop assistants fought their way to sit at this till and at least one, after six years of infertility, conceived immediately having gained this seat. One shop assistant was recorded as saying 'we avoid it like the plague'. In its report, the *Today* programme did not mention whether there is a nearby monastery.

I am not at all sure that firmly planning when to start a family really makes much sense for most people. On the other hand, whenever people do have their first baby, life will become different in a way which is difficult to imagine completely and certainly cannot be fully anticipated. Looking after a new person brings extraordinary responsibilities and is, apart from anything else, a most maturing influence. These responsibilities are not that easy to predict, and therefore nobody can plan so perfectly that they will be able to cope with all the changes in their lives. Having a baby changes how both partners think about themselves. It may alter a relationship with one's own parents. It can also change a couple's views about some friendships and will almost certainly (at least temporarily) change one's interests in life, focus ambitions and alter one's attitude to a job. No matter how consciously the decision to have a baby is taken, this time of major change in life is not something which can be entirely planned.

Making the decision

Most couples will want to discuss having a baby well before the event. Some books advise you to work out how starting a family will change your lives, and some couples even map out how they will divide responsibility for the baby. However, to my mind, this does not make much sense before pregnancy. Inevitably, a special bond between mother and baby develops. A mother's closeness to her child after birth and the act of breastfeeding are both facts of life that inevitably exclude the man to some extent. Following the birth of a child, men will take on a role that cannot be entirely predicted.

I am reasonably certain about at least one thing. Getting pregnant is generally a poor way of cementing a failing relationship. Of the unhappy infertile women who come to me, desperate to have treatment to get pregnant, many tell me that they are terrified that their relationship with their partner cannot survive unless they have a baby. It is sad to see how often women believe that, by having a baby, they will prevent their partners leaving them. In my experience, having a baby doesn't help. I have seen people go through endless treatments to get pregnant – surgery and test-tube baby treatment included – but the final success often heralds the beginning of the break-up of their relationship.

Happiness is not ensured by having children. Children can be wonderful but they also disrupt your life, are often noisy, frequently messy, involve extra work and cost money. They also usually reduce a woman's opportunities for independence outside the home and interrupt many promising careers. Certainly, one thing that may need to be discussed is the subject of money. A good rule is to reckon with a reduced income, and perhaps it is a sensible idea to plan one's finances before getting pregnant.

Leaving it until later

Some women put off having a baby because they are developing a career. Having a baby can be a great intrusion if one is in a fulfilling or exacting job. If one is just getting established, having a baby may interrupt an important chance of success. In addition, many women find it very difficult to get back to full-time work after having children. For all these reasons, most obstetricians have the impression that, more than ever before, they are looking after more women in their late thirties or even early forties who are having their first babies.

Other women may conceive later in childbearing life for quite different reasons. An older woman may not be able to get satisfying work that is equal to her enthusiasm or abilities. Some people in this situation choose to get pregnant as a kind of consolation, but this may be a short-term solution to the problem, once the child starts going to school. I also meet many couples who delay having a child till later on in life because one or the other had an unhappy childhood. A feeling of not wishing to perpetuate a bad experience makes many women and men reluctant to commence a family until very late.

Another reason why people suddenly decide to start a pregnancy at a later age may be that they simply cannot imagine the future without children. This can be a remarkably sudden feeling which women especially experience in their later thirties. This may happen after years of feeling quite remote from any idea of a pregnancy, particularly if life with a new partner is contemplated.

Mary, a determined and talented journalist, decided at twenty-eight that she never wanted children. Her feeling of certainty was absolute, and her husband also had no desire to have children. To Mary the very idea of pregnancy was off-putting, but most contraceptive methods caused her unpleasant side-effects. Eventually she decided on sterilisation, but because she was still so relatively young, she could find no gynaecologist prepared to go along with the idea. Convinced that what she did with her own body was her affair and after reading an advertisement in a newspaper, she turned up at a private family planning agency and requested sterilisation. After a five-minute consultation, she entered a private clinic for an overnight stay. Clips were placed across both of her Fallopian tubes in a fifteen-minute operation, fortunately a relatively reversible procedure.

Thirteen years later, when Mary was forty-one and divorced, she fell in love with another man. She felt that she would be failing him totally if she could not offer him children. She could not bring herself to tell him that her tubes had been clipped. Although strongly advised to tell him the truth beforehand, she went through a major operation to have the sterilisation reversed without his being informed about why the surgery was being done. She gave all the nurses in the hospital strict instructions not to let the cat out of the bag. So far, sadly, she has not conceived.

In Chapter 5, we look at some of the physical implications of embarking on pregnancy later in life.

Controlling fertility

Many people are worried that their method of contraception might make it difficult to conceive after stopping. Is there any evidence for this?

THE ORAL CONTRACEPTIVE PILL

'The pill' is frequently blamed for making people infertile. However, studies by the Royal College of General Practitioners in Britain show that 80 per cent of all women who have never had a baby, and ninety per cent of those who have, will have conceived within one year of stopping the pill. This is exactly the same proportion of pregnancies found in those who have not used contraception previously. Nor does the length of time that a woman has been on the pill matter.

Some women (about 1 per cent) do stop having periods after coming off the pill, and consequently they have difficulty conceiving afterwards, but this percentage is exactly the same as would be expected to be found in an equivalent population not taking the pill. However, just to be safe, most doctors would agree that women having very infrequent periods may be better off not using the pill.

STARTING A PREGNANCY AFTER STOPPING THE PILL

Ovulation may occur immediately on stopping the pill. Alternatively, several weeks may elapse before the normal menstrual cycle restarts. A woman who is in the rare group (1 per cent) of people whose periods do not return within three months should visit her family doctor. Treatment is usually very simple, requiring a 'fertility pill' (see p. 167). A few women may need stronger drugs, given by injection, to stimulate their ovaries more vigorously (see p. 171).

Some women, on the other hand, appear to become more fertile on stopping the pill. This so-called 'rebound fertility' is somewhat disputed, but there does seem to be limited evidence for it. Certainly, in our laboratories, when rats were given the hormones contained in the pill – which were then stopped abruptly – they were more than normally fertile immediately afterwards, tending to have more babies in a litter. This effect was only temporary.

Because coming off the pill tends to have a somewhat unpredictable effect on when ovulation restarts, most obstetricians think it wise for women to avoid getting pregnant immediately after ceasing oral contraception. Whilst no harm occurs when this does happen, many doctors advise waiting until at least two periods have occurred before trying to conceive. This is simply because it makes accurate dating of when the pregnancy started easier. However, now that we have very precise ways of measuring the early progress of pregnancy with ultrasound (see p. 148), I personally think that this really doesn't matter.

One further point. Some recent reports have suggested that a miscarriage is a bit more likely in women who conceive immediately after stopping oral contraceptives. The evidence for this is, to my mind, totally unconvincing. Miscarriage is an extremely common event and it is probable that the group of women who participated in these studies were monitored so closely that early miscarriages, which normally might well have gone unnoticed (at least by a doctor), were recorded and presumed to be an effect of the pill.

THE INTRAUTERINE DEVICE (IUD) –
THE 'COIL'

There is no particular reason not to try to become pregnant as soon as an IUD, or coil, is removed. In recent years, however, there has been something of a question mark over fertility after coil removal. In general, fertility does not seem to be impaired after removal; a large study in the United States in 1968 showed that 60 per cent of women conceived within three months, and that 85 per cent had conceived within a year. These figures were also borne out by a study by the World Health Organization, which looked at women from many different countries; the percentage of women getting pregnant was about that expected in a normal population. However, it may be unwise to use the coil if one has never been pregnant. There is recent growing evidence that a number of young women, mostly those who have never been pregnant, are at greater risk of pelvic infection if they wear a coil. This kind of information is difficult to evaluate, because pelvic infections are a bit more common if a woman has had a number of different sexual partners. While it is possible that 'coil-users' may be only at extra risk because they may have more sexual partners than average, it is probably sensible not to use the IUD if you have never been pregnant previously.

INJECTABLE HORMONES

Some publicity has been given recently to trials of contraceptive hormones given by injection. The hormones involved are mostly a form of synthetic progesterone (such as Depo–Provera) and are used by comparatively few women. The advantages of this method of contraception are the relative safety of these injections and the fact that one injection will last for several months – very satisfactory for the forgetful sort. This kind of drug has not found wide acceptance because, in spite of its undoubted safety, there is some risk of weight gain and irregular bleeding, and because quite a few women only return to normal fertility several months after ceasing the injections. These hormones are therefore not very suitable if one might want to get pregnant at a particular time.

Timing a pregnancy

People have not just recently become interested in controlling family size and in timing pregnancy. On the contrary, contraception is an extremely ancient practice. The Petri papyrus, dating from around 1850 BC, describes how, in Egypt, crocodile dung was made into a paste and inserted into the vagina. The Ebers papyrus, probably dating from 1550 BC, contains a particularly interesting prescription: 'Beginning of the recipes made for women in order to cause no conception for one year, two years or three years: Take tips of acacia. Mix with a measure of honey, moisten lint therewith and insert in her vulva.' Of course, we have no idea whether this worked, but it is curious that the tips of the acacia plant contain gum arabic, and this, when moist and fermented, liberates lactic acid – a substance widely used in many modern spermicides.

Researchers have come up with some interesting evidence that contraception may have worked satisfactorily before the present century. For example, one study of Europe's ruling families showed that there was a steady decline in their birth rate. Under scrutiny were the births to aristocrats in their first and only marriages. It was found that, from 1500 to the beginning of the twentieth century, the number of children fell from a high of more than six (in about 1570) to about three.

Another study, which examined the birth rates of 1900 British aristocratic families, showed a similar trend: the mean number of sons fell from 5.6 during the years 1730–1779 to 2.4 during the period 1880–1939. As the only available methods of contraception were either abstention from sex or the withdrawal method (and, in the absence of contraception, abortion), it is

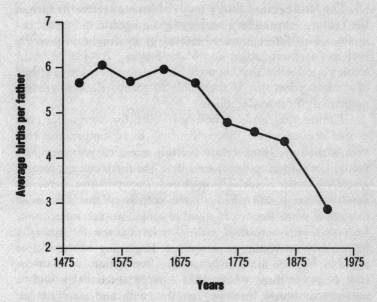

The declining birth-rates in European noble families. This evidence suggests that they deliberately limited the number of their children after 1700, possibly using interrupted coitus. There is not likely to be an economic reason for the decreasing fertility of the aristocracy.

likely that these aristocrats chose to withdraw. It seems unlikely, after all, that the average English duke would abstain . . .

THE FERTILE PERIOD AND
TEMPERATURE CHARTING

The fertile period is, of course, the time in the menstrual cycle when conception is most likely. Remarkably, it was only in the twentieth century that people generally recognised the existence of a fertile period. The extraordinary studies of Dr Raciborski of Paris in the 1840s have already been described (*see* p. 17), but they did not gain wide acceptance.

The fertile period finally received attention after the turn of this century – not to help people to get pregnant, but rather as a method of contraception, advocated by birth control pioneers such as Margaret Sanger and Marie Stopes.[8] Avoidance of the fertile period – the 'rhythm method' – has been the only method of contraception that is acceptable to many religious groups, particularly Roman Catholics.

Timing the fertile period was virtually impossible until people became aware that a woman's body temperature rose after ovulation. Temperature charting was first suggested as a method of contraception in 1904 by a South African gynaecologist, Dr Van der Velde. The method for temperature charting is described on p. 134. While I am convinced that this is an extremely poor way for an infertile couple to time intercourse, I accept that this method may have limited use for normally fertile couples trying to achieve a pregnancy as rapidly as possible. Nevertheless, studies in the United States show that at least 20 per cent of women with a temperature that would be considered normal 'ovulatory' are not, in fact, ovulating at all. And my impression is that at least another 20 per cent of women with a virtually flat or irregular temperature chart are ovulating normally.

CERVICAL MUCUS EXAMINATION

As we have seen, cervical mucus changes in character during the menstrual cycle. Shortly after the period stops, the cervix begins to make watery mucus in increasing amounts. At the time of ovulation, this mucus production is at its peak and the mucus is at its most penetrable by sperm. It looks and feels

[8] Remarkably, that great pioneer of contraceptive methods, Marie Stopes, to whom modern women should be truly grateful, was brought up to be entirely ignorant of the functioning of her own body. Some time after her marriage, she suspected that her marriage had not been consummated. She had to go to the local public library before she could confirm she was still a virgin; her marriage was eventually annulled in 1916.

rather like the uncooked white of an egg. Immediately after ovulation, when a woman is no longer fertile, the mucus thickens and then shortly afterwards dries up almost completely.

Some women produce so much mucus at ovulation that it tends to run out of the vagina like a watery discharge; others produce very little. A woman who tends to have a clear watery discharge immediately before ovulation may have an obvious, simple external sign that tells her when she is ovulating.

Unfortunately, these signs are very vague in practice. Any vaginal infection (and this is extremely common), or any semen or other secretions from sexual activity, make it very hard to tell when the fertile period has arrived. Moreover, many women who are ovulating perfectly normally never produce enough mucus to make external assessment of this sort possible.

URINE TESTS FOR LH

It is possible now to buy a kit from the local chemist which helps establish when ovulation is about to occur. This is a simple urine test, containing a chemical which changes colour if plenty of the LH hormone is being produced (see p. 000). On the face of it, this seems a remarkable advance as it should mean that couples can more easily decide when they want a pregnancy. Unfortunately, these kits are by no means all that the advertisements would have us believe. Several manufacturers are responsible for different versions of basically the same test and much glossy advertising and slick packaging has gone into them. I regret to say that I think they are almost useless as they have many serious drawbacks:

● The tests are expensive, costing perhaps £20–30 per month.

● Many people find it difficult to get the right colour change, and they get worried unnecessarily because they think they are not ovulating.

● The tests measure LH, the message to the ovary to ovulate. The ovary may get the signal from the brain but it may not

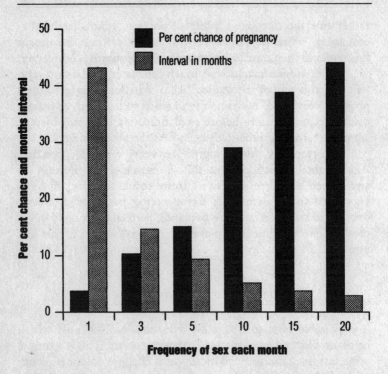

respond. This is like a friend telephoning you at home – you may not be in to lift the receiver. This kit, in effect, merely shows that a signal went down the line, not whether it was picked up or acted upon.

● Some women have high, fluctuating LH levels which give false positive readings. They could think they are ovulating when they are not.

● The manufacturers imply that timing intercourse increases the likelihood of getting pregnant. This is debatable and seems exploitative.

● Timing intercourse so precisely is emotionally destructive and can damage a relationship. In my view, it should be used with extreme caution by most couples. It may be more satisfactory for a normally fertile couple, but then a normally fertile

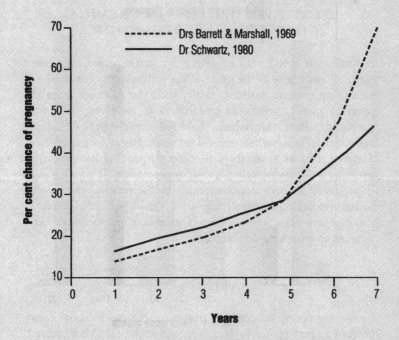

The chance of a normal couple having a baby depends very much on how often they have sex. Daily sex does not weaken the sperm; on the contrary, all the evidence suggests that fertility is improved with frequent intercourse. With sex once a month, the chance of a pregnancy is only 3 per cent, and the average time a couple would have to wait before conception is 42 months. With sex twenty times a month, the chance of conception each month is over 40 per cent.

couple will hardly ever need to go to these lengths to get the woman pregnant. Consequently, I think these tests should probably be used only in very specific circumstances, and then probably under sensitive medical guidance.

RECENT POSSIBILITIES IN CHEMICAL DETECTION OF OVULATION

A somewhat better way to detect the fertile period may be to measure oestrogen in the urine. This will have the advantage of measuring ovarian activity, rather than the message from the pituitary gland. Australian researchers are working on a very simple 'dip-stick' test, which could measure the peak of soluble oestrogen in urine which should occur shortly before ovulation. Another area of research is to deter impending ovulation by studying a substance called guaiacol peroxidase. This substance is produced in high concentrations in the cervical mucus just before ovulation. A simple 'dip-stick' could be briefly placed in the vagina by the woman herself, enabling her to detect early signs of approaching ovulation.

MAKING LOVE

I now can reveal how to get pregnant. No matter how many books you read on the subject, you will seldom find it discussed. If you are unlucky enough to be having difficulty in conceiving, you will usually not be told the real secret. The truth is that, the more often you make love, the more likely a pregnancy. The more infrequently you have sex, the less likely you are to conceive.

There are numerous myths surrounding conception. Two of the most common are:
● if you are having trouble getting pregnant, you should make love less frequently so that the sperm have a chance to get strong, more copious and/or more active;
● pregnancy is not happening because one is not pinpointing the moment of ovulation.

I know of no evidence to support either of those statements. There is, however, abundant evidence that frequency of sexual intercourse is directly related to chances of conception, and that the timing of intercourse only needs to be loosely over the fertile part of the month.

Various recent studies have shown the advantages of frequent intercourse and its effects on conception. One, published in 1983, showed that couples having sex once a month between the woman's periods took an average of 43 months to conceive; with sex 3 times a month, the average delay in conception was 15 months; 10 times a month, the average delay was 5 months; and if a couple had sex more than 15 times a month, the average length of time it took to conceive was 3.5 months.

A very good friend of mine – whose name I cannot publish because she would be besieged for all kinds of advice – had great difficulty getting pregnant for a second time. She is a very determined lady. After many months of failing to conceive even though she and her husband tried to time intercourse for the 'fertile period', she finally insisted that her unfortunate partner made love to her at least once every night for a month. She says he was a bit exhausted after this (which, incidentally, he denies completely – though he certainly played less football), but her daughter was born nine months later.

CHAPTER THREE

Discovering You Are Pregnant

I do not know whether this is wishful thinking, but some women seem certain that they can tell when they are pregnant virtually from the moment of conception. This is difficult to prove, and seems rather unlikely. It is very doubtful that such a small structure could make enough hormones at this stage of development in amounts sufficiently great to be detected by the woman herself. The embryo is so tiny in the first week or so of its life that it is invisible to the naked eye. Moreover, it does not enter the uterus until about the fifth day after ovulation. We do know, however, that, although the embryo is free-floating at this stage and in no way attached to its mother, it soon begins to produce various chemical signals, including hormones, which tell the lining of the uterus to prepare for its implantation. The embryo, still microscopic, starts to attach itself there about a week or so after fertilisation – that is, about twenty-one or twenty-two days after the start of the last period in a woman with an average menstrual cycle. Implantation is accompanied by quite a complex reaction, so it is just possible that this fierce little chemical fire is detectable very early on.

Symptoms that are suggestive of pregnancy

Even before there is a strong suspicion of pregnancy, some of the following symptoms may be experienced.

TIREDNESS

Many women notice that they are much more tired than normal. Very often this means being sleepy in the morning or feeling very thick-headed in the evening. Carrying out routine tasks often seems to involve remarkable effort. This tiredness may be felt very early on, and it frequently disappears later on in pregnancy, some time around the twelfth week. What causes this tiredness and lethargy is difficult to explain, but it is certainly true that an early developing pregnancy consumes some of the body's energy sources. Interestingly, a few women feel much more alert in early pregnancy.

NAUSEA AND VOMITING

Feeling nauseated, or actually being sick, is one of the most common symptoms of pregnancy. Classically, this feeling is at its most unpleasant first thing in the morning, and is made worse by rapid changes in posture – for example, getting out of bed. However, it is almost equally common to feel sick at other times of day, particularly in the evening. Nausea can often be controlled to some extent by regularly taking small bites to eat, particularly food with a relatively high carbohydrate content – for example, dry biscuits.

Generally, nausea occurs slightly later than tiredness. Feeling sick may be due to the outpouring of pregnancy hormone (human chorionic gonadotrophin), which starts to increase about sixteen days after ovulation.

BREAST TENDERNESS

This occurs frequently and may be felt very early on in pregnancy. Some women certainly experience this as the first definite sign each time they become pregnant. Although breast tenderness is also extremely common towards the start of a period, very often women only experience it when they are pregnant. Sometimes, the first sign may be nipples which feel very tingly or particularly sensitive. I also know of some women whose first symptom is that their bras don't fit – though typically, breast enlargement is a much later sign, by which time most know for certain that they are expecting.

CHANGES IN APPETITE

These are very common. Some women become exceptionally hungry in early pregnancy. Others feel like eating unusual foods. The husband of one of my friends always knows when his wife is pregnant because she starts getting out of bed at 5.00 a.m. to make peanut butter sandwiches – something that, normally, she can't stand. Some women develop a peculiar taste in their mouths, which they often describe as 'metallic'. A few women have an overwhelming desire to eat certain non-foods – a condition known as *pica*. I have known patients who ate plaster from kitchen walls and lumps of coal.[9]

URINARY FREQUENCY

It is quite common for women in early pregnancy to feel the need to empty their bladders much more frequently. This can occur well before the time that the uterus starts to enlarge, so it cannot be due to the bladder being moved from its normal position. Having to go to the toilet frequently may be due to a high level of the hormone progesterone in the blood, which tends to relax the gut and bladder muscles of the body.

[9] Dr Fournier of Paris in his sixty-volume *Dictionnaire des sciences médicales*, published in 1812, describes a pregnant woman who developed something of an appetite for her husband's blood, cutting him gently while he lay beside her and sucking the wounds.

MOOD SWINGS, HEADACHES, WEIGHT CHANGES

Some women just feel different – either elated or depressed – in very early pregnancy. It is quite common to be unexpectedly tearful, just like before a period. Headache, or even migraine, is a very unpleasant symptom. Those who are unfortunate enough to suffer from these symptoms in early pregnancy may take some consolation to know that they tend to disappear completely by the twelfth or thirteenth week.

Some women also lose or gain an unusual amount of weight in the first three weeks of pregnancy.

NO PERIOD

Of course, this is the most important symptom of pregnancy. A person normally having regular periods whose period is late by more than four days is most likely to be pregnant. Loss of a period (amenorrhoea) can be due to a number of causes, but in women up to the age of forty it is most commonly caused by being pregnant.

Sometimes an unusual period may occur. About one-third of women have some kind of bleeding in early pregnancy at or around the time when their periods would normally occur. A period which is much lighter than normal, or much shorter, or accompanied by fewer symptoms of discomfort are all quite typical of those that occur in early pregnancy.[10]

[10] Although cessation of menstruation is the most important sign of pregnancy, it is not necessarily reliable. There is a peculiar condition called 'pseudocyesis' – false pregnancy – when women stop having periods and complain of feeling pregnant. The most famous case of pseudocyesis must be that of Mary I of England. A Catholic heir was much needed by her husband Philip of Spain. Mary apparently prayed constantly for a pregnancy, otherwise the succession would go to her sister Elizabeth. Finally her periods stopped, her breasts enlarged and the nipples became discoloured, she had violent vomiting, and an increasing abdomen; apparently she even spent time making baby clothes. At the end of the ninth month she had labour pains, and the bells of

Testing for pregnancy

Until comparatively recently, testing for pregnancy required a hospital laboratory. The most common test, until the 1960s, involved injecting the woman's urine into a rabbit or a toad and waiting many hours before inspecting the ovaries. Nowadays – and good news for toads and rabbits – most family doctors, family planning clinics or chemist's shops will arrange a rapid chemical test. This detects the pregnancy hormone human chorionic gonadotrophin (HCG), which is produced by the embryo within seven days of fertilisation and is detectable in urine within two and a half weeks or so. There is also a rapid and highly sensitive blood test for HCG which can be done by many hospitals. This can detect a pregnancy within twelve days of fertilisation, before a period is even missed. However, this test is not widely used because it is relatively costly.

Many women now like to test themselves for an early pregnancy. There are several excellent kits on the market which can be bought from the chemist. Although most are very accurate, none is quite as good as a test done in a hospital laboratory.

● *Predictor.* This is widely available at around £7.90 per kit. It is very accurate and can detect pregnancy, in some cases, as early as two days after a missed period. A sample of urine should be collected immediately upon getting out of bed in the morning, as this is when it will be most concentrated. This should be mixed with a reagent in a little tube, according to the instructions supplied with the kit. A special plastic indicator is inserted into the urine for a variable amount of time (thirty minutes if the period is two days late; five minutes if it is more

London were rung to announce the new heir. People rushed to St Paul's Cathedral to hear the Archbishop of Canterbury describe the child and bless him. Finally her pains ceased and the Queen had 'violent hysterics'. Subsequently, of course, Philip of Spain departed and the succession went to Elizabeth I.

than five days late). The tip of the indicator will turn pink if there is a pregnancy. Two points to remember: the indicator should not be left in for longer than forty-five minutes, as the result may be inaccurate. Also, the test is designed for normal room temperature, and may not be quite so reliable in a freezing room.

● *Clearblue*. This kit is available at around £6.95 for two pregnancy tests in one kit. It claims to be able to diagnose pregnancy within a day of a missed period. With this test one urinates over the end of a plastic sampler, which is then inserted into two plastic wells in turn for ten minutes. It is a bit more complicated than the Predictor test, and can involve more time. As soon as the sampler has been washed under a running tap of cold water, it can be examined it to see if it has turned deep blue. This indicates pregnancy. If it is only light blue, a test is needed again in a few days. Points to remember: cold water should be used to wash the indicator which must be examined immediately afterwards; the colour on the indicator is matched under a good light with that supplied on a chart; it is only accurate with concentrated, 'first thing in the morning' urine.

● *Clearblue One Step*. A more rapid test has recently been marketed which consists of only one step. It costs about £8.35 for two tests. A small absorbent sampler is placed in the stream of urine, holding it there for five seconds. The end of the sampler is then secured in its plastic cap and the two windows in the side of the sampler are examined. With pregnancy, a thin blue line appears in the bigger window. This test is also said to be capable of detecting pregnancy on the first day of a missed period. One point to remember: the tip of the sampler must be held downwards in the urine stream. I like this test. One of my patients recently sent me her plastic sampler with the blue line in the window to prove she was pregnant after some tubal surgery I had done. She also sent me a rose on St Valentine's Day, which worried her husband.

All these tests are reputable but, of course, not cheap. All may be inaccurate if a woman is having hormone injections containing HCG which may be used by a few doctors for those prone to miscarriage, or those having test-tube baby treatment.

In these situations, a false positive result can occur. False negative results are not that unknown, so women who continue to feel pregnant after repeating a negative home test should certainly see the doctor.

When to see the doctor

In general, women who have had no difficulty conceiving or no paticular gynaecological problems in the past have no need to rush to see their doctor. Those who have had infertility treatment or previous miscarriages or an ectopic pregnancy (*see* Chapter 13), should make an appointment as soon as they think they may be pregnant. This is to check that the pregnancy is developing normally and is in the right place. Those who have had any previous difficulties in conceiving may need early ultrasound examination (*see* p. 148). This is partly to date the early pregnancy accurately and to provide reassurance that the baby is growing normally. Women who have had any serious medical condition – such as diabetes, heart disease, asthma or a kidney complaint – should also make early antenatal appointments at a hospital clinic.

CHAPTER FOUR

Can You Select the Sex of Your Baby?

Since earliest times, people have been fascinated about the possibility of being able to detect the sex of an expected baby. The ancients often believed that it is possible to influence a baby's sex, and even nowadays some people seem quite convinced that various bits of hocus-pocus may make some magical difference.

In Chapter 1 we saw that each sperm and egg contain twenty-three chromosomes. When the sperm and egg fuse, the resulting embryo cell contains forty-six chromosomes, made up into twenty-three pairs. This total is kept in all cells which divide from the first embryonic cell. One pair of chromosomes, which are rather smaller than the others, contain (among many others) the genes for determining sex. The female sex chromosome is called the X-chromosome, the male the Y-chromosome. All mature eggs contain only an X-chromosome. Sperm, on the other hand, may have either a Y-chromosome or an X-chromosome. When the sperm enters the egg, the embryo which results will either have XX-chromosomes, in which case it will be female, or XY-chromosomes, in which case it will be male. There must be at least one X-chromosome in every mammal's cell (except the sperm cells). This carries other essential genes which are necessary for all animal life. Because the sperm may contain either an X- or Y-chromosome, it is the man who indirectly dictates the sex of the baby. There are rare occasions when an individual can be born with more than two sex chromosomes. Multiple copies of the X-chromosome do not always cause a person to be abnormal. Multiple copies of the Y-chromosome, for example XYY, are usually associated with aggressive criminal behaviour.

Curiously, there are actually more male babies than females. In an average population, for every 100 girls born, there are 106 boys. The reason for this is not entirely clear. As far as we know, the number of Y-bearing sperm in a man's semen is equal to the number of X-bearing sperm. Consequently, it is thought that an equal number of female embryos are conceived, but that more are lost because they do not implant properly in the uterus.

Ancient customs, old beliefs

Many ancient peoples, coming from quite different origins, had remarkably similar beliefs about the factors affecting a child's sex. Boys were favoured by the ancient Chinese who often felt that the appearance of a woman's face in pregnancy gave a clue to the sex of the baby. An Egyptian manuscript of 2200 BC tells that a pregnant woman with a greenish hue to her face is certain to give birth to a son. In ancient India, physicians suggested that if a pregnant woman had a fresh, clear complexion and a rounded abdomen, if her right eye was bigger than her left, or if her left breast showed more activity than her right, this foretold a boy. These beliefs were also prevalent in ancient Greece and Rome. The Greeks also though that boys moved earlier in pregnancy, a folk belief that prevails to this day. Hippocrates thought that stronger seed from the man produced boys – and, as we shall see, perhaps he was not quite so far from the truth. However, he also thought that a mother who developed freckles was more likely to produce girls.

Many ancients, including Hippocrates, thought the side on which the man and woman lay during and after intercourse was important – right for a boy, left for a girl – a belief which persisted even in this country until the twentieth century. It was thought that a fusion of the 'humours' from the right testicle and the right side of the abdomen would form a boy. Anaxagoras actually proposed the tying off of the left testicle to produce only boys. Remarkably, some French noblemen in the seventeenth century were actually persuaded to undergo this form of half-castration to ensure an heir, despite the fact that, 2,000 years earlier, Aristotle (384–322 BC) had pointed out that men with only one testicle were capable of producing either boys or girls. These French counts were either ill read, well hung or desperate. Other Frenchmen of the time, being less bold, merely favoured pinching their left groin at the crucial moment of pleasure.

The timing of intercourse was also thought to be important by some Greek philosophers. Empedocles (c.490–430 BC), who is credited with founding the first medical school, suggested that males could be produced by having sex during menstruation, because he thought ovulation occurred then. Aristotle, who showed so much remarkable intuition about so many things and was an undoubted master biologist, felt that the timing of intercourse was not important in determining the sex of a baby as it was possible to have twins of different sexes. He also (rightly) argued that the sex of a child depended on the man.

That great collection of Jewish writing, the Talmud, which dates from about the third century AD, has many references to methods for sex selection. In one Talmudic tractate called Niddah, Rabbi Isaac states: 'If a woman emits her semen first, she bears a male child, if the man emits his semen first she bears a female child.' ('Emitting semen' most likely refers to orgasm.) Rabbi Kattina boasted, 'I could make all my children males', implying that he was able to restrain himself during intercourse. Rashi, a famous Jewish commentator of the twelfth century, suggested that having a male child is the Talmudic reward for having assured that one's wife has her orgasm first. He advised a husband to have intercourse twice in rapid succession, assuming that that way a woman would be bound to have an orgasm at least once before her husband. In another part of the Talmud, it says that it is a vain thing to pray specifically for either a boy or girl; interesting that ethical arguments for and against sex selection were considered so long ago.

Why select the baby's sex?

Various reasons have been given for people wanting to select the sex of their babies. Studies conducted in recent years show that even in apparently civilised societies such as ours, boys are more desired than girls. In one American study, 1,500 married women under the age of forty were questioned, and twice as many wanted boys as wanted girls. The reasons they gave for preferring a boy were: to please their husband, to carry on the family name and to provide a companion for their husband. Another study in the US in 1970 showed that the majority of American women wanted two children, with a boy first.

In countries with high population growth and low economic development, boys are much more in demand. This is partly due to the fact that boys are more likely to become breadwinners and will be capable of supporting their parents when they are old and infirm. Two doctors, working in Poona, India, quote a farmer from the Punjab: 'You were trying to convince me as a poor man who could not support a family in 1960 that I should have no more sons. Now, you see, I have six sons and two daughters and I sit at home at leisure. They are grown up and bring me money. Now, you see, because of my large family, I am a rich man.' A lucky man, indeed.

It seems that there was huge aversion to female births in ancient civilisations. It was no accident that Pharaoh found that the most damaging thing he could do to the Hebrews was to throw all first-born male children into the Nile. That way, of course, he destroyed the providers and soldiers. As recently as 1885, the traveller Vambery, returning from Asia Minor, quoted the Turks:

> If a daughter is born to thee,
> Better she should not live,
> Better she should not be born, or, if born,
> Better the funeral feast with the birth.

Some modern authors appear to believe that sex selection could answer urgent world problems of overcrowding. They claim that the ability to choose the sex of one's child, combined with adequate contraception, would ensure a male and thus reduce the need for larger families – and, by implication, unwanted girls. The moral aspect of these arguments will be dealt with later.

Perhaps the only clearly valid reason for sex selection is for couples who are at risk of transmitting a severe disease which is sex-linked: that is, only boys or (more rarely) only girls will suffer the effects of such a disease. Perhaps the best known of these is haemophilia; another is a very grave form of muscular dystrophy; and some types of severe mental defect are also X-linked, only affecting boys. There are, in all, about 300 diseases which are sex-linked; most, but not all, of them affect only boys. In this situation, it seems perfectly reasonable to try to ensure that any child that is born is female, if possible. Interestingly, this approach would not eliminate sex-linked diseases, as they are generally carried on the X-chromosome. Carriers of these diseases are girls, and they, though not affected themselves, could pass on the disease to half of the boys to whom they gave birth.

Sex selection has only been sanctioned in Britain when it is clear that a child might die of a sex-linked disorder. There was a fierce debate about this quite recently in 1990, during the passage of parliamentary legislation on human embryology (*see* Chapter 15). Just before this debate, Baroness Warnock, the much respected Cambridge philosopher and chairman of the Warnock Committee (Government Enquiry into Human Embryology), was quoted as saying that she could see nothing wrong with peers of the realm ensuring that they had a male child to carry on the hereditary peerage.[11] There was not much

---

[11] This extraordinary statement was completely in keeping with the demeanour of many other noble members of the House of Lords. During discussions on the rights and wrongs of insemination with donor sperm, many Scottish hereditary peers seemed far more worried about how this important social issue

sympathy for this observation, though I have to say that I can see little wrong in using sex selection, if it were possible, to help families who persistently have had repeated pregnancies resulting in children of only one sex. My personal view is not shared by most medical ethics committees, and unless there is a change in viewpoint, the method of sex selection described at the end of this chapter will only be offered for couples carrying severe gene defects in their families.

Factors said to influence a baby's sex

STRESS

It has been claimed that stress is capable of altering the chance of having a girl. Professor Hampe, a German, writing in 1862, noted that poor people in a particular town during hard times were more likely to have boys. Dr Ploss, an Austrian, noted in 1882 that, given unfavourable conditions, male births were more likely. Several authors have since claimed that following various European wars, there was an increase in the number of male births.

WATER SUPPLIES AND ENVIRONMENTAL POLLUTION

Dr Lyster made many studies of the different rates of birth of males and females in various populations under different environmental conditions in the 1960s and 1970s. He claimed that, in Australia, male births were reduced some 320 days after changes in the water supply, brought about by heavy storms. He also thought that a variety of environmental pollutants

---

might affect the laws of inheritance and succession, than any other aspect of the legislation on fertilisation and embryology.

affected births, arsenic in the atmosphere causing an increase of males, births near iron and steel works being more likely to be female. Dr Lyster was a wonderful enthusiast. He spent much of his later professional life in the semi-darkness of hospital basements (where birth records are usually kept) trying to amass statistical evidence to support his controversial observations. They are not altogether accepted.

SEASONAL INCIDENCE

In the last century, several authors claimed that more females were born in spring, more boys in autumn. The German, Dr Dusing, felt that the increase in sexual activity, due to a rise in temperature, might play a part. I credit Dr Dusing with the first experiment to attempt to select sex in 1890. Because he felt that greater sex drive in the male produced a female baby (a widely held belief, dating back, as we have seen, to the Talmud), he tried an experiment in thirty cattle. He describes how he encouraged a bull to have intercourse in rapid succession with many different cows in order to weaken it. He then led the exhausted bull to a cow which was well nourished, well rested and sex-starved. According to Dusing, because the cow enjoyed the subsequent conjugal relations with its tired mate, it produced a bull-calf. Conversely, Dusing claimed to have produced heifers by feeding a bull with plenty of good grass and isolating it from cows until it was absolutely 'rearing to go'. Perhaps this is where we get the phrase 'at the end of one's tether'. In the meantime, its prospective mate had sex repeatedly with a castrated bull (so that it could not conceive) until the cow 'no longer had any sexual desire'. It was then mated with the well-fed but sexually frustrated bull. This procedure invariably produced cow-calves. Dr Dusing does not state whether he tried this approach in people.

WHAT ABOUT CROCODILES AND ALLIGATORS?

Sex selection in some reptiles is of great interest to biologists. Studies in these creatures certainly provide an example of how environmental conditions may play a crucial role in affecting the sex of offspring. Dr Ferguson, of Oxford University, has recently reported on his experiments. If an alligator's egg is incubated at 86°F (30°C) during certain times of development after fertilisation, all the embryos are female. If incubated at 91.4°F (33°C), then all the embryos are male. If incubated at temperatures in between, then a varying proportion of male and female offspring are produced. In nature, because most eggs are incubated at around 86°F (30°C), there are six times the number of females to males. Incidentally, these temperature changes also induce changes in the size of the animal and its skin colour. Dr Ferguson and his colleagues have actually switched eggs, held at different temperatures, between nests of these voracious creatures to see what happens. I have this happy picture of these dedicated scientists on tip-toes tripping around sandy beaches, avoiding snapping cavernous jaws, in the interests of scientific endeavour. Alligators do not have special X- and Y-chromosomes apparently, having possibly lost them during the evolutionary process. In their case it may be that the gene which determines sex is on other chromosomes and that this gene is regulated by the environment. The concept is of great interest because it does suggest that changes in surroundings or chemicals may be of profound genetic importance in different species.

Sex selection methods

TIMING INTERCOURSE

Very many writers, since earliest times, have felt that the timing of intercourse (in relation to the time of ovulation) may affect the sex of a child. Various instructions are given in different literary sources.

The earliest detailed description I can find, which readers might like to try out, comes from an old Hindu source, the *Susrutas Ayur Vedas*. Assuming you want a boy, you must separate from your man three days after your period begins. A special, rich diet is recommended. On the fourth day of menstruation, dress in your best clothes and look at your husband. You should now avoid sex for one month, until your next period starts. Anoint yourself with oil on the fourth, sixth, tenth and twelfth nights of your mentrual cycle and make love. If you want a girl, try sex on the fifth, seventh, ninth and eleventh days of your cycle.

Some writers have claimed, until surprisingly recently, that women ovulate from alternate ovaries each month. This observation led Dr Dupuy (1888) to advise couples to count the number of menstrual periods since the last confinement. Those who wanted a child of the opposite sex from the previous pregnancy were advised to have sex only in the odd-numbered months following the last delivery (that is, to have a baby girl after a baby boy was born in December, intercourse should occur in January, March and so on). Looking back on the dates of my own children's birthdays, I found this theory to be totally proved.

Many modern authors have claimed that having sex close to ovulation is more likely to produce a girl. One study in Jerusalem, among very orthodox Jewish women who avoid sex for the first seven days after their periods, showed that, in 3,658 births, 53.3 per cent were male if intercourse occurred two days before ovulation, 49.3 per cent were male if conceived on the day of ovulation and 65.5 per cent male if conceived two days later. This difference was said to be just statistically significant.

This method apparently worked very well for Mrs Monteith Erskine, the wife of a Scottish MP, who in 1925 wrote a very earnest book, *Sex at Choice*, explaining how to get boys. She herself had conceived one girl and four boys precisely as she wished, depositing her secret formula for timing with her bankers in London. She also described how:

Nature intended women to produce more boys than girls, and that, with this end in view:

1. She provided the girl-child with more male ova in her right organ ovary than female ova in her left.

2. She rendered easier the fertilisation of the right-side ovary . . .

3. She made the right ovary and tube larger than the left and provided more seminal fluid for them to carry.

Presumably Mr Monteith Erskine was a Conservative MP.

EVIDENCE FROM STUDIES ON ARTIFICIAL INSEMINATION

More recently, various clinics performing artificial insemination using donor semen have had the opportunity to analyse their results following insemination at various times close to ovulation. A well-controlled study in the United States showed that the sex of 1,188 children, each conceived after a single insemination, could not have been predicted by the time in the menstrual cycle when insemination was done. More recently, two doctors in London have found no evidence of a preponderance of boys or girls related to the timing of ovulation. They did find, however, that women who took clomiphene, the fertility drug, and who then had insemination, appeared more likely to have girls. We have looked at women taking clomiphene in our hospital, and have not found any change in the normal sex ratio.

It is very likely, as we shall see later, that all these observed differences are due purely to chance. When the first test-tube babies were born, there was a definite increase in the number of girls. The first test-tube baby was Louise Brown and she had a sister a few years later, also conceived by in vitro fertilisation treatment. Since then, however, the proportion of girls to boys has evened out. In our clinic, 52 per cent of these babies have been boys – what would be expected in a normal, untreated population.

VAGINAL DOUCHING

Since about 1930, several doctors have claimed (without any hard evidence at all) that sperm with a Y-chromosome prefer an alkaline environment, while X-carrying sperm prefer acid. This curious notion has persisted and is still commended by people practising fringe medicine. They prescribe douching the vagina with a solution of bicarbonate of soda for a boy, or lemon juice or vinegar for a girl. Apparently this should be done about fifteen minutes before sexual intercourse. Try this if you must; my feeling is that your vinegar would be better employed on a green salad.

SHORTENING THE ODDS

Dr Cedric Vear of Australia and Dr Landrum Shettles of the United States (both fairly controversial figures) have advised similar régimes, a combination of some of the techniques I have already mentioned, and have claimed that these work. If you have a good sense of humour, you might like to try to:

For a boy
1. Abstain from sex from menstruation until ovulation has occurred.
2. Douche with 5 g of soda in a pint (0.5 litre) of water, fifteen minutes before sex.
3. Have sex with the man behind, and with deep penetration at ejaculation.
4. Ensure that female orgasm occurs before ejaculation.
5. Stop intercourse the moment the man ejaculates.
6. Repeat this rigmarole 2–3 times in the next twenty-four hours.

For a girl
1. Douche with 1–2 tablespoons of vinegar in a pint (0.5 litre) of water, before sex.

2.   Have frequent sex in the 7–10 days before ovulation.
3.   Have no further sex during the twenty-four hours before ovulation is expected.
4.   Have sex face-to-face, with only very shallow penetration.
5.   Stop sex after ejaculation.
6.   Ensure that female orgasm does not occur.

Using these techniques, Dr Vear had ten successes in ten pregnancies – but it took him seven years in an obstetric practice which was delivering over 200 babies each year. It is hardly surprising that he had so few volunteers when you think about it – a messy douche fifteen minutes before intercourse, deep rear-entry sex hopefully with a good female orgasm, avoid sex completely for two weeks beforehand and then have it four times in rapid succession. I think he was quite lucky to find ten couples, but how did he make sure they did it properly?

DIET

It has been suggested for well over 100 years that dietary factors can influence the sex of your child. Dr Schenk from Hamburg, writing in the last century, describes a woman who had five boys and who then developed diabetes; in her sixth and seventh pregnancies, she had a girl. Dr Schenk considered that her deteriorating body metabolism led her to have girls, and he 'confirmed' this observation by studying the urine of many other patients – those that contained sugar were prone to give birth to girls. He therefore tried deliberately to reduce sugar in the urine with special diets to produce boys. One of his colleagues, in writing up these studies, remarked: 'As is well known, Schenk was not altogether fortunate in his experiments.'

Some authors have held that the mineral content of a woman's food can influence the sex of her child. Most of this work comes from France, a country where cuisine is noted for its powers. For a boy, you need to have a diet rich in potassium with added salt. Such a diet might include sausage, meat, potatoes, beans, artichokes, peaches, apricots and bananas. For a girl, these foods should be avoided and more calcium with magnesium is needed. Suitable foods include dairy products, eggs, grapefruit, radishes, turnips and greens. A book by Labro and Papa (Photobooks, Bristol, 1984) describes the dietary requirements in detail. They do not look particularly appetising to me and I am a little surprised that French pride allowed publication.

THE MAN COULD CHANGE HIS JOB

One study suggests that fighter pilots have a 59.3 per cent chance of a boy, transport pilots 62.5 per cent and airfield ground staff 60 per cent. Commercial underwater divers and anaesthetists are reported to have more girls. In practice, although various claims have been made, the variations in ratio can easily be attributed to chance.

SEPARATING AND SELECTING X- OR Y-BEARING SPERM

It has been known for some time that male sperm are different from female sperm, and various scientists have tried hard to separate them. The idea is that, following separation, only sperm of the 'right' sex might be inseminated into the woman's vagina. The X-chromosome is a bit bigger than the Y-chromosome, and therefore a female sperm might be expected to weigh very slightly more. A great deal of attention has been given to this, and several methods of separating male and female sperm depend on this rather obscure piece of biology. I calculate that a single sperm probably weighs less than 10 picograms (that is, ten million millionths of a gram). Regrettably the Y-chromosome is almost the smallest identifiable structure in the sperm head, and at a liberal estimate an X-carrying sperm probably weighs no more than about 3 per cent more than a Y-carrying sperm. I am not sure I can work out the precise difference, but it doesn't seem much, not when dealing with such a minuscule object as a sperm.

Various laboratory methods for separation have been tried. They are all very similar, and all have similar deficiencies. The most publicised involves spinning semen in a centrifuge, having first suspended it in various liquids which have either a particular viscosity ('pourability'), causing more resistance to the sperm, or molecules of a certain size, which act as a kind of filter. Dr Ericsson of Sausalito, California, uses this method to separate Y-sperm, saying that 'It's like making them run the Boston marathon with overshoes on.' According to *Time* magazine, each clinic in the United States which uses his technique pays him $15,000 in franchise fees. However, Dr Sandra Carson, a reproduction expert at the University of Tennessee in Memphis, was unable to validate the method. Dr Ericsson's California car number plate is: X OR Y.

From time to time, there are press reports from Japan about sex selection. Both *Time* magazine and *New Scientist* recently carried stories about methods to separate X- and Y-bearing sperm to produce either girls or boys. Dr Iizuka of Keio University, Tokyo, has apparently used the technique to produce girls in all six patients who volunteered – a number too small to justify any statistically verifiable efficacy. Nevertheless, the results brought a storm of criticism from Japanese ethicists and were extensively published in newspapers there. Apparently this techique has also been used by a Dr Sugiyama in 120 cases: 24 women conceived, and in 22 cases, girls were subsequently born.

Dr Sugiyama's success rate – 22 out of 24 conceptions – is certainly large enough to confirm a definite effect not due to chance. Consequently, many Western scientists and doctors find it extremely surprising that, years later, the only accounts of this technique have been in the popular press and it has not been refereed by a medical or scientific journal. Until that happens, we shall remain sceptical.

DOES SPERM SEPARATION REALLY WORK?

Methods to separate sperm are not new. Indeed, an electrical method was first described by a Dr Schroeder in Germany in 1932 and, since that time, it has been 'rediscovered' by several authors. However, there are a number of criteria which have to be met before one can say that there is a genuine and reliable method for sex selection.

● *There must be controlled clinical trials.* This means that a given treatment, for which claims are made, has to be allocated to patients on a random basis in advance of treatment and the results assessed independently. So far, no method of sex selection has been subjected to controlled trials.

● *The observed difference between male or female births must be proved to be not due to chance.* Few methods of sex selection clearly demonstrate that the results they have produced are not due to coincidence. Hardly any of the authors have used a proper control group (i.e. couples giving birth who have not undergone any special treatment) to act as a simultaneous comparison, and most report very small numbers. For example, Dmowski, who used a layering technique in 1979, said that six out of eight couples had boys after his work. This ratio is likely to be due purely to chance. It has been calculated, using detailed mathematical formulae, that at least nine out of ten couples would have to achieve the desired sex before it could be assumed that the observed difference is not due to chance.

● *The method should be capable of such scrutiny that a reputable medical journal will publish the results, after independent peer review.* Authors of a substantial number of so-called scientific papers on the subject have not risked presenting their work to proper journals. In many cases, claims have only been made in the popular press such as *Time* magazine.

● *Others must be able to reproduce the method both in animals and humans.* Very few, if any, of the methods of sex selection have been found to be repeatable by independent scientists or doctors.

What also impresses me about 'sex selection' is that many of the methods have been promoted by fringe practitioners, and that some people conducting sex selection clinics seem to be making considerable sums of money.

Very recently (1992) considerable publicity has been given to a GP working somewhere in east London who, it is claimed, has set up a clinic offering sex selection. He is said to filter male sperm from the semen, subsequently inseminating it into the vagina of women who pay around £200 each cycle. This could ensure him large profits. The chance of conception in a single insemination cycle is around 15 per cent, so a couple having this treatment would need to attend five times to have an evens chance of pregnancy. I know of no properly published data which prove his success rate in producing children of the desired sex. To my mind, this doctor, whilst possibly making a good deal of money, may be running considerable risks. Unless he has been properly trained in reproductive medicine, he presumably risks being struck from the Register for offering services which are 'beyond his competence'. Moreover, only one abnormal child needs to be conceived for him to be liable for massive legal damages. Such practitioners are probably best avoided.

A woman came to see me, complaining of infertility. Initially, she told me that she had been trying to get pregnant for two years, without success. However, she then revealed that she had already had three children, and that she had had no difficulty in conceiving any of them. There was nothing in her medical history to suggest why she should have become infertile, and her husband was in good health, she said. I was puzzled about her strange demeanour. When I hinted that I would much prefer to do tests on both her and her husband, she most reluctantly brought him to see me. It transpired that they had not had intercourse for two years. Eventually, I learned that all three of their children were girls and that they wanted a boy. Apparently they had been trying to conceive a boy by visiting an American practitioner. On three occasions they had flown from London to New York, where a doctor had inseminated her with her husband's sperm, having first treated it by a method of sperm separation. Each insemination cost $500 – a hefty sum a few years ago, considering that the laboratory work lasted thirty minutes and the insemination took five minutes. I suggested her 'infertility' (which distressed her very greatly) was simply due to lack of having intercourse and that she might be better off trying to conceive naturally.

I can suggest an even better money-spinner for an enterprising young doctor. Human gullibility is such that it should be possible to offer a treatment for sex selection, with a full money-back guarantee. The doctor carries out treatment at $500 a time. If the baby is the wrong sex, a full refund would be made. This should offer a very attractive income, on the grounds that 50 per cent of the time the doctor would get things right.

ABORTION

Clearly, one way of ensuring a baby of the 'right' sex is produced is to screen each pregnancy by chorion villus sampling or amniocentesis (*see* pp. 294–6). If the baby is not the desired girl or boy, termination of the pregnancy can then be carried out. From time to time, gynaecologists in Britain are asked to carry out screening and (if desired) abortion by patients who simply want to select the sex of their children for purely social reasons. I do not know of any colleague who is prepared to do this, and most people view the idea with alarm and repugnance.

This does not always appear to be the establishment view in other countries. In 1982, in India, two physicians in Amritsar advertised amniocentesis at sixteen weeks' pregnancy to detect daughters, and offered abortions. After protests by women's groups, the health minister announced that such abortions were not allowed. However, surprisingly, the issue did not end there, and it seems that the Indian Goverment, which sees overpopulation as the country's main problem, does not actively discourage the practice.[12] In India, it appears that successful research on

[12] There is good evidence of regular female infanticide, practised to this day in Rajasthan, in Rajput, India, using opium or suffocation by sand. The problem,

how to conceive males would be welcome. A review of attitudes to this problem was published in 1986 by the International Sociological Association.

It might be thought that, in Western countries, there would be very serious concern at the idea of aborting a foetus of the 'wrong' sex. However, one study done by psychologists in the United States showed that up to 40 per cent of the population did not consider it particularly worrying and men were less concerned than women.

COMMERCIAL KITS FOR SEX SELECTION

It seems that all aspects of human reproduction are very interesting to the media. A recent programme on British television discussed a sex selection kit, on sale in American supermarkets for just $40. If you want a boy, you buy the blue box; if a girl is desired, the pink one is purchased. Each kit contains a thermometer (value $2.50) and some litmus paper (probable value 50 cents). It also contains information about various positions you should adopt during sexual intercourse (value incalculable). The television presenter concluded: 'It's a bit worrying that this is on the market. It is not available in Britain.' She could have added that there is absolutely no evidence that it works.

According to the *Guardian*, one American company marketing a kit called 'Gender Choice' (price $45) claims to have tested it with 6,000 couples with an 85 per cent success rate. The company, Procare Industries, based in Colorado, hoped to export it to Britain in 1986. It involves the use of daily vaginal swabs to predict the ovulation pattern; how this might help sex selection is not clear, but the president of the company, a certain Robert Marsik, said that the secret lies in the 'precise timing and method of intercourse'. It is interesting that there have been no

according to Pamela Nowicka (*Observer*, 2.8.92) is the high cost of a girl's dowry. Late abortion is also used here; across the country there are notices up: 'Spend 600 rupees now, save 50,000 rupees later.'

validated medical trials of this product (published in peer review journals). So far, in spite of threats, this product has not hit the UK market as far as I know. Perhaps Mr Marsik became aware that there is some medical evidence to show that delaying conception around the time of ovulation might theoretically lead to a woman having a chromosomally defective child. Maybe he was worried about lawsuits.

Argument for and against sex selection

Many sociologists and psychologists have debated the consequences of sex selection. Their conclusions are as follows:

ADVANTAGES	DISADVANTAGES
Avoids sex-linked disease	Might benefit rich people only
Boys/girls might feel especially 'wanted'	Boys/girls might feel 'unwanted'
Balance of two-child family	Imbalance of sexes in population
Reduction in population in under-developed countries	Increase in conflict between sexes
Increases human genetic controls	Risk of eugenics (i.e. 'master race')
	Possible abuse by the state

The main argument against sex selection, and the one most frequently presented, is that there would automatically be a preponderance of boys in the population as most people would rather have boys than girls. However, various studies have shown that, at least in developed countries, the preference for boys is very slight. Most people questioned have maintained that they do not care which sex their children are. About 4 per cent would prefer a boy and about 3 per cent a girl. It is very unlikely that this could make much difference, if any, to the ratio of girls to boys in the population at large.

So is reliable sex selection really possible?

The answer is yes. Our research at Hammersmith Hospital suggests that a comparatively reliable method of sex selection is now available.

The method involves using test-tube baby treatment to collect eggs and fertilise them outside the body. One single cell, quite invisible to the naked eye, is removed from the embryo while it is growing in the test tube, three days after fertilisation. The removed cell is immediately destroyed and its DNA content analysed, while the embryo is kept in culture. Using a recently discovered method of gene amplication, powerful techniques are used to identify whether or not the single cell contains a Y-chromosome. This test is so exquisitely sensitive that laboratory workers of the opposite sex to the embryo, by coughing carelessly or brushing cells from their fingertips, could introduce their own DNA into the solutions which are used and this could give a false result. However, so far, using absolutely strict controls, the sexing of each embryo has been correct in every case except one. So far six babies have been born to families who previously had lost a child afflicted with a sex-linked genetic disorder; a few more healthy babies are on the way. One woman conceived with a foetus of the 'wrong' sex, and elected to have the pregnancy terminated because there was a serious risk of sex-linked haemophilia. This technique is complex and expensive, and because of this it is inappropriate to be used for frivolous reasons.

I must emphasise that this technique has only been developed to help couples who are at risk of giving birth to children with serious or fatal sex-linked diseases. There is no intention to offer this treatment for 'social' reasons.

CHAPTER FIVE

Late Motherhood

Recently, there has been much interest in childbearing at an 'advanced' age. Complex medical treatments have made it increasingly possible for women to get pregnant in their late thirties and early forties. Unfortunately, these treatments have far too frequently raised unrealistic expectations. In this chapter, I examine the biological limits, why we become decreasingly fertile and how these limits might be safely or unsafely manipulated.

Many of the women whom I see as patients are trying to get pregnant in their late reproductive years. Nearly all of them know that age is a bar to fertility; most show great interest in what is the biological time-limit for conception. The oldest known mother to give birth in Britain (where the dates can be verified) was Mrs Elizabeth Pearce, from Southampton. She had a son in February 1916, when she was just a month over fifty-four years old. Such advanced age at childbirth would appear to be excessively rare because the only other case in this century of a British woman giving birth at a similar age is that of Mrs Wilson of Eccles, who had a daughter in 1936 when she was fifty-four, or possibly, fifty-five years old.[13] There are reports of older women giving birth, but it is likely that many of them are cover stories for younger relatives and for illegitimate grandchildren. It seems that advanced age was possibly less of a bar to fertility in ancient times, though of course it is

[13] She was born in Wolverhampton on 11 November, but for some reason there is confusion about whether she was born in 1881 or 1882.

impossible now to verify some remarkable tales. Pliny mentions Cornelia of the Serpios family in Rome in his *Historiae naturalis*. She is said to have borne a son at sixty years, calling him Volusius Saturninus. In the *Philosophical Transactions of the Royal Society of London* (1722), Dr Wallace speaks of a woman from the Orkney Isles having a child past sixty.

> My favourite case, reported in the French medical literature, *L'Union médicale de Paris*, 1881, is that of a widow of Garches, a village just beyond Saint Cloud, then outside Paris. She was seventy years old and liked to indulge herself in a few bottles of wine. On one occasion, after an unusually prolonged libation of *vin rouge* she found herself unable to walk home and sat by the roadside awaiting sobriety. There she was found by a young man from the same region who knew her, and who offered to help her homewards. By the time the house was reached, night was well advanced and she invited him to stay overnight. One thing led to another, and finding her more than affable, he stopped for four nights. The result of these kindnesses was an ensuing pregnancy for Madame.

Whilst pregnancy in women in their fifties is obviously very rare, I find it very curious that we doctors regard pregnancy in a woman over the age of thirty as abnormal. Yet when I was in training, any woman having her first baby when she was over thirty was called an 'elderly primigravida'. This term seems to imply that the unfortunate woman is in her dotage and needs special mollycoddling to coax her through what is an appallingly dangerous time. It is perfectly true, of course, that biologically speaking the best time to get pregnant is between the ages of twenty and twenty-five. However, in my own antenatal clinic the great majority of women are clearly 'elderly', with an average age of over thirty-five. This is because most of my own patients are rather infertile and usually have been trying to get pregnant for many years. They are none the worse off for that, and as they are all unfortunately younger than I am, I can hardly regard them as elderly.

Why are people waiting so long to have babies?

Perhaps the most common reason is simply that both men and women do not like to commit themselves early in life. In past years, people got married at a very young (perhaps too young) age. The changing pattern of Western society has meant that many men and women put off a firm commitment until much later, preferring to rear children when they are more sure of ther own future. I think that, in many ways, we have become a very responsible society; I get the strong impression that a great number of men and women defer having children until they are certain of themselves as people, until they are fully mature.

Of course, while nowadays relatively secure and easy contraception has encouraged more people to delay childbearing, it is clear that a major factor is the question of career. Far more women than ever before work for a living. The gradual liberation of and increasing opportunities for women have also meant that they are faced with a dilemma. Many patients I see have decided to establish themselves in a career first, before trying for a baby, and then panic suddenly, seeking help to have a baby 'before it is too late'. Increasingly frequently we find that women over thirty who are having a baby for the first time are not married.

How increasing age affects fertility

It is surprisingly difficult to prove that slightly older people, and especially women in their later thirties or early forties, are much less fertile than younger ones. Clearly, though, there is a gradual decline in human fertility with age and in women, this decline starts well before the menopause. This decrease is seen in all populations, in many different countries. In order to understand the way this opinion can be arrived at, and what its

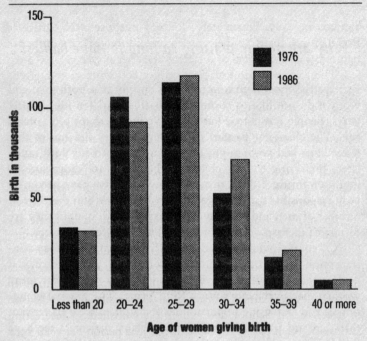

The statistics for births in England and Wales in 1976 and 1986.

consequences are for the average couple, let us look at some statistics.

If we examine official records taken from all women resident in England and Wales in 1975, we find that there were about 690,000 pregnancies. This figure rose steadily over the years until, in 1985, there were 797,000 pregnancies. Incidentally, the number of pregnancies outside wedlock[14] – 160,000 in 1975 – rose to 283,000 in 1985. Of course, not all these pregnancies resulted in children being born and many more occurred but miscarried, but these are not recorded in official statistics; in addition 106,000, were terminated by legal abortion in 1975 and

[14] This high percentage of all pregnancies conceived in 1985 (35 per cent – a rise of 12 per cent out of wedlock in ten years) says a good deal about changing attitudes in society. Partnership without marriage is now clearly the norm, and I think it a good reason for doctors to be prepared to treat infertile couples who are not legally married.

142,000 in 1985. Fortunately, for our purposes, the Office of Population Census Studies gives a breakdown of the number of babies born to mothers of different ages (*see* p. 78).

These figures show us that only 4,800 women in England and Wales gave birth at or after the age of forty, both in 1976 and 1986. Although there was generally a trend for women to have babies at an older age – more women delivered a baby between the ages of twenty-nine and thirty-nine in 1986 than in 1976 – there was no increase in the number of babies born to women over 40. This suggests that, despite social pressures and trends, it was not possible for women to alter their basic lack of fertility after a certain age.

It could be argued that the birth rates for present-day England and Wales are not truly representative of basic fertility because so many women nowadays use some form of contraception. For this reason, I have chosen to look at some statistics from populations who had no known access to birth control. In 1985 Professor Trussell of Princeton University and Dr Wilson of the London School of Economics published an interesting study of British parish registers during the period between 1500 and 1849. In all, they looked at sixteen different parishes, deliberately sampling a cross-section of the population of England to include rural villages, market towns, cities and industrial areas. They were examining how many women, married at different ages, did not subsequently produce children. Their data are important for three reasons. First, contraception was not in use during the period in question. Second, it is most unlikely that abortion would have any major influence on their results. Third, by careful reading of baptismal, marriage and burial registers, they were able to include only women who had 'completed unions' – that is, those who remained married until the end of their reproductive period, i.e. would or could have been having intercourse. Trussell and Wilson's results are shown in the graph on page 80.

This fascinating study tells us a good deal about human fertility. We can see that only about 7 per cent of women who married at a very young age remained infertile but at least one-third of women who were married at the age of thirty-five did

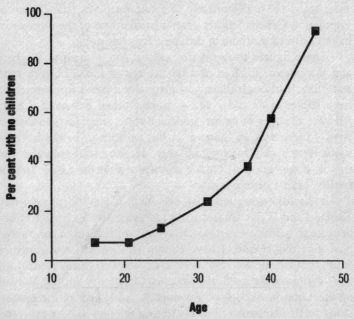

The chance of older women not having a baby.

not give birth. Nearly 60 per cent of women married at forty had no children, and there was only the tiniest chance of a pregnancy after the age of forty-four. This data, though fascinating, may however be seriously flawed. A number of these marriages were probably never consummated – there is good historical evidence that failure to consummate marriage was commoner before television was invented. Also, I presume that even in remote parts of rural England, villagers would understand the withdrawal method of contraception, a practice known about since biblical times.

Is the phenomenon of decreasing fertility simply a British one? The answer is almost certainly no. Similar trends are seen in other human populations. Of particular interest are the Hutterite women. The Hutterites are an ultra-religious, inbred, Protestant sect living in the United States and Canada. They have been repeatedly studied by anthropologists, sociologists

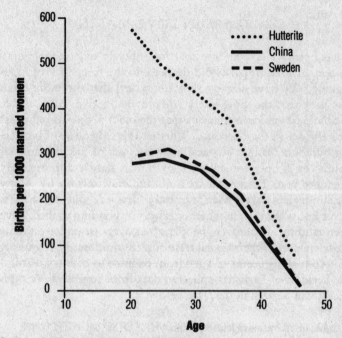

Declining fertility in three different populations.

and others for a number of reasons, one of the main ones being the Hutterites' high natural fertility. They seem to be more fertile than almost any other group of humans.

Why are older women so infertile?

Like so many things about human reproduction, it is not fully understood why older women are so infertile. It is likely that several possibilities may contribute to the problem.

DECREASE IN LOVE-MAKING

It has been widely thought that infertility in older people may be due, at least in part, to a decrease in the frequency of love-making. We have already seen (*see* p. 47) that the more often you have sex, the more likely you are to conceive. All available sociological evidence suggests that the older people are, the less sexually active they become. Whether this is because of increasing boredom, failing physical prowess, lack of the first flush of youth, or simply too much television is hardly appropriately discussed here. Firm evidence is not too easy to come by. Many questionnaires have been earnestly devised, but researchers never know for certain whether people responding to them have been truthful. Moreover, people often over- or under-estimate the frequency of their sexual relations. In addition, the frequency of love-making seems to vary from country to country. Professor Leridon of Paris has collected data from several studies; his results can be seen in the table below.

AGE OF WOMEN AND MONTHLY FREQUENCY OF SEXUAL INTERCOURSE
(MARRIED WOMEN LIVING WITH HUSBAND ONLY)

AGE	US	FRANCE	PUNJAB	BRITAIN	AUSTRALIA
16–20	11.0	–	8.5	9.9	17.2
21–24	10.1	10.9	8.5	8.2	12.0
25–29	9.0	10.9	8.5	6.9	10.0
30–34	8.0	–	5.2	5.3	9.2
35–39	6.8	7.8	3.0	5.5	8.0
40–44	5.9	7.8	2.2	*	6.8
over 45	–	3.2	1.5	*	5

* There are no accurate statistics available for British women.

Those who thought that the French were the sexiest nation in the world are clearly wrong. The British do no more than live up to other people's expectations. Australian women come up trumps, or perhaps they just boast a lot. Unfortunately, I know of no data suggesting whether Australian women are more fertile than others; however, Americans appear to be more sexually active than the British and this could explain why they seem to be more fertile. These figures confirm that sexual activity decreases with age.

ABNORMAL MENSTRUAL CYCLES

As women get older, they do not ovulate as regularly or as frequently. There are two good studies – one carried out by Dr Dorling in 1969 and the other by Dr Vollman in 1977 – which confirm this (see below).

FREQUENCY OF IRREGULAR MENSTRUAL CYCLES IN OLDER WOMEN

APPROXIMATE AGE	ABNORMAL CYCLES (Dorling's data) %	ABNORMAL CYCLES (Vollman's data) %
30–35	16	13
36–40	19	11
41–45	30	16
46–50	51	30

These figures, while demonstrating that a sizeable minority of women have menstrual problems, also show that many have perfectly good cycles well into their late forties. Clearly, then, failure to ovulate is by no means the whole reason for failure to conceive in this age group. This is important because so many of the women of this age who come to me complaining of infertility are convinced that, because they are having normal cycles and are ovulating, they should be able to get pregnant easily. In fact, other statistics show that, on average, biological infertility commences ten years before the menopause (when periods stop or become irregular) in British women. What this

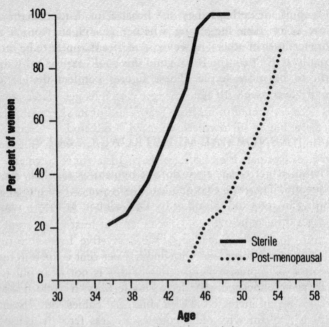

On average, biological sterility occurs about ten years before a women stops seeing her periods.

means is that a woman has to put up with periods for an average of ten years even though she has ceased to be fertile.

DECREASE IN MALE FERTILITY

A third reason is perhaps due to male infertility. There is quite good evidence that men, too, become increasingly infertile with age. Clearly, older women will generally be married to older men, and if it is true that male fertility decreases with age, this could partially account for the fact that older women conceive less readily.

Of course, male fertility does not decline as sharply as does female fertility – there is no menopause, as such. Moreover, it is true that many men remain fertile until very late in life. One of our husbands at Hammersmith fathered quadruplets at the age of seventy.[15] Pablo Picasso fathered a child at eighty. One of the best examples of male fertility in old age is Baron Baravicino de Capelis of the Tyrol, who died in 1770. He married his fourth wife when he was eighty-four and had eight children by her; she was pregnant with the last when he died. His generative ability has been attributed to his diet – eggs, no meat, sweet tea and a cordial made to his own secret recipe. I did find the recipe for Baron Baravicino's recipe in an old book somewhere, but, very sadly, cannot pass it on because I have mislaid it somewhere.

There is a serious side to the fertility of older men. Some recent research in Canada suggests that, compared with younger men, those over forty-five years old produce far more sperm which are defective. It seems likely that at least 16 per cent of sperm from male Canadians over forty-five have abnormal chromosomes, compared with about 4 per cent in men in their twenties. The precise significance of this is not clear but it is likely to be associated with decreasing fertility. It could also just account for an increased risk of abnormal babies, but certainly helps to explain why older couples are less fertile because in most instances women tend to marry men rather older than themselves.

INCREASED RISK OF MISCARRIAGE AND GENETIC DEFECTS

Older women have a greatly increased chance of miscarriage. Many of these lost pregnancies undoubtedly occur so soon after conception that women do not know that they have even been pregnant. Obviously, this may be a factor in the low fertility of older women. (For a full discussion of miscarriage, see Chapter 13).

Miscarriage at any age is extremely common. A study

---

[15] We were hounded by the press for undertaking fertility treatment in this couple, but having seen this happy family grow up over some eight years, I have no doubt that the treatment was justified.

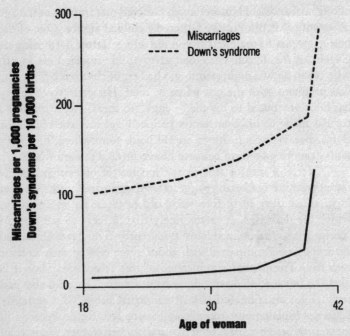

The rising incidence of miscarriage with age exactly parallels the rising incidence of Down's sydrome. This is evidence that faulty eggs are likely to be a common cause.

carried out in 1962 suggests that at least 23 per cent of all pregnancies of more than four weeks end in miscarriage. Another piece of research in 1970 suggested that 49 per cent of all fertilised eggs perish before full-time delivery. Results from patients having test-tube baby treatment (IVF) in our clinic suggest that the first figure may be a little high; we find that less than 15 per cent of test-tube pregnancies end in miscarriage once they have survived as long as four weeks. However, the situation following this treatment may be different from what happens after natural fertilisation; after all, following IVF only the best embryos are transferred to the womb. It is likely that at least 60 per cent of fertilised eggs do not make viable babies. What is clear is that older women have a much greater risk of miscarriage.

We do not know why the risk of miscarriage increases with age. Probably it is because an older woman produces less healthy eggs. These eggs have been held in her ovaries for a long time; indeed, they have been there since before her birth. Since that time, the eggs have been in arrested stage of development, and have been exposed to many potentially adverse infuences in the environment. Eggs which have become damaged are more likely to produce damaged embryos if fertilised. This could well explain, at least in part, why older women are more likely to miscarry and also why certain genetic defects are more common in babies conceived by them.

We know that about 40–60 per cent of all miscarried foetuses show some chromosomal defect on examination, the majority being due to having one extra chromosome, medically called *trisomy*. It is worth remembering that Down's syndrome (or mongolism) is particularly common in pregnancies in older women. This defect is a trisomy, which fits well with this theory. What is even more interesting is that the increased likelihood of Down's syndrome with age closely parallels the rising chance of miscarriage. This, I think, gives us an important clue as to the cause of miscarriage in older women.

PROBLEMS IN THE UTERUS

Failure to get pregnant at a later age may also be partly due to problems in the uterus (womb), which in older women contains more fibrous tissue and less muscle, and is also more apt to contain a fibroid (*see* p. 89) or have some adenomyosis (*see* pp. 108–9). In addition, the endometrium, the lining of the uterus, is more likely to be abnormal and less able to help an embryo to implant properly.

It has also been suggested that the blood supply of the uterus is not as good in older women. The evidence for this is not yet very compelling, and more research is required. However, it could be one reason why infertility is more likely and miscarriage more common.

Are there extra risks in becoming pregnant after thirty-five?

It is important to realise that being pregnant when one is older than average carries no very great risks. The great majority of 'older women', when they are fortunate enough to get pregnant, have a perfectly healthy and happy pregnancy, a normal delivery and a bouncing, normal baby. Moreover, many abnormalities associated with age can be screened for in the foetus (*see* Chapter 14). The risks of pregnancy in older women are nowadays also greatly diminished as antenatal care gets better. In general, the risks are:

GENERAL MEDICAL AILMENTS

All men and women are prone to ill health with age. All of us tend to be fitter at twenty than at thirty, and fitter at thirty than at forty. Apart from general physical fitness and well-being, general health problems also increase slightly as we reach the age of forty. The most important of these are changes in our blood vessels. Unfortunately, perhaps partly because of diet and environment, we humans are prone to diseases of the circulation system as we get older.

In pregnancy, the most important problem is an increased risk of high blood pressure. A rise in blood pressure, when it occurs, is more likely in mid-pregnancy and can affect the baby. Babies of mothers with high blood pressure are more likely to have problems or to be small and of low birthweight. Consequently, women with high blood pressure (hypertension) may require much more rest in pregnancy, and, quite frequently, even hospital admission before delivery. Raised blood pressure is more likely if there is a family history of this problem (about which one can do nothing) or in those who smoke, are overweight, are under stress or drink too much alcohol (something can definitely be done about these).

Two other quite common circulatory problems which are a bit more likely in older pregnant women are varicose veins and blood clots in veins (venous thrombosis). Neither of these is particularly serious. Varicose veins can be unsightly and make the legs ache, but usually all that is needed is more rest than usual and support tights. Venous thromboses are more common after delivery than before it, and cause pain and soreness. Support tights are also often helpful with this complaint, and occasionally drugs to thin the blood and stop it clotting readily (anti-coagulants) may be needed. These drugs can be given quite safely and without the risk of bleeding excessively during the delivery of the baby.

Other medical problems which occur slightly more frequently in pregnancy are diabetes, gallstones, bronchitis, certain rare types of anaemia and, very infrequently, low thyroid gland activity. None of these is common (except possibly diabetes) and certainly none is sufficiently serious to warrant any real concern about getting pregnant. The risk of diabetes naturally worries older women who are pregnant, especially if there is a family history of the disease. This worry is natural, but most diabetic states in pregnancy are simply and easily controlled with diet alone and, occasionally, bedrest.

FIBROIDS

One common problem in women over thirty-five years old is fibroids. People with fibroids are less fertile than average. It has been calculated that, by the time they are forty years old, about one-third of all women have some fibroids, benign swellings in the uterus (see p. 108). They may be only the size of a grape, or grow bigger than a melon. Fibroids very seldom cause symptoms in non-pregnant women and during pregnancy they rarely cause difficulties. Occasionally they may be associated with miscarriage, and in exceptional circumstances may make a normal delivery less likely and delivery by Caesarean section may be indicated.

MISCARRIAGE AND STILLBIRTH '

The most important risk is very early loss of the pregnancy. As we have seen, miscarriage is much more common in older women. The reasons are not entirely clear, but are probably the same reasons why women over forty are so infertile. Older women have eggs of less good quality in their ovaries, many of which may result in defective embryos. These embryos may survive very early pregnancy but could not survive in the outside world. The uterine environment is also less satisfactory with advancing years, and the uterus may simply reject the newly formed embryo. Finally, older women are generally married to older men and, as we have seen, older men produce sperm with a higher percentage of abnormalities.

All these risks have to be seen in context. Even younger women in their thirties have a significantly greater risk than women in their twenties, and nobody in their right mind would suggest to a thirty-five-year-old woman that she is too old for childbearing. Most women in their forties who face the greatest risk come from very poor backgrounds, tend to have poor nutrition, cannot look after their health, are sometimes overweight and often smoke heavily. Very often they have had many pregnancies previously, and this, too, can sap their wellbeing. It is therefore very important to get the real risk into sensible perspective; it is much smaller than many friends, relatives, professionals – particularly well-meaning midwives and doctors – will have us believe!

GENETIC DEFECTS

Just as miscarriage is more probable because of defective eggs, genetic defects are also a little more common in the babies of older women. The most important of these problems is the chromosomal defect Down's syndrome. Down's syndrome is usually caused by there being three copies (instead of the normal pair) of chromosome 21. About 60 per cent of cases of Down's syndrome follow fertilisation of abnormal eggs carrying extra chromosomes. This condition is also more common in women who have already conceived a Down's syndrome baby. The increasing risk of conceiving a baby with Down's syndrome is shown in the chart below.

Having three copies of one chromosome is called trisomy. Trisomy of other chromosomes is also a bit more likely in older women – in particular, trisomy of chromosomes 13 to 18 and, more rarely, trisomy of sex chromosomes. Down's syndrome is especially important because it accounts for a large proportion of all mentally retarded infants (32 per cent in Britain); it is, by far, the most common cause. Unfortunately, children with Down's syndrome also frequently have other defects (such as heart problems) and are very prone to infection; as a result, they have a greatly shortened life expectancy. The implications of all this are discussed in Chapter 14. Suffice it to say, Down's syndrome – as indeed all other foetal defects associated with age – can be reliably detected early in pregnancy.

RISK OF CHROMOSOME ABNORMALITIES IN BABIES OF OLDER WOMEN

AGE OF WOMAN	RISK OF DOWN'S SYNDROME	ANY CHROMOSOME DEFECT
20	1 in 2000	
25	1 in 1205	1 in 527
30	1 in 885	1 in 476
35	1 in 365	1 in 204
37	1 in 225	
38	1 in 180	
39	1 in 140	
40	1 in 109	1 in 73
41	1 in 85	
42	1 in 70	
43	1 in 50	
44	1 in 40	
45	1 in 32	1 in 23

For discussion of the pros and cons of screening for these defects, and the special tests that can be done, *see* Chapter 14.

SMALLER BABIES

Older women are a little more prone to having babies of a lower than average birthweight. This probably reflects the fact that they tend to have higher blood pressure, and that the uterus has a poorer blood flow. For this reason, most obstetricians tend to want to see older patients more frequently during pregnancy and may recommend rather more frequent ultrasound scanning. If the baby is growing at a slower pace than normal, the advice may be to come into hospital for extra bedrest and for pregnancy monitoring.

PROBLEMS DURING LABOUR

Some older patients may have a bit more difficulty with delivery. My own feeling is that these difficulties are often greatly exaggerated. Positive thinking is better than negatively assuming that trouble at delivery is inevitable. It is true to say that those in the older age group will probably not be as used to physical exercise and, as a result, pushing the baby out may be more of an effort. However, mental attitude is all-important.

Fortunately, nowadays, there is no extra risk to the baby if assistance with delivery is required because of maternal fatigue. If the baby is also getting tired or distressed, a Caesarean section may be recommended. This may come as a shock initially, but it is worth remembering that this is only advised when the doctors need to make certain that the baby will be born with the least risk. Modern practice at many hospitals allows a Caesarean operation under local (epidural) anaesthesia, which means that mothers may be awake to experience the birth. In addition, it is increasingly common for partners to be together during a Caesarean section, and many couples find this a great comfort. Those who are interested in this idea should certainly consider asking if this may be possible.

WILL I FEEL TOO OLD?

Perhaps the biggest problem that older women face is being afraid of feeling old. Attendance at an antenatal clinic can mean being surrounded by women fifteen or more years younger than oneself. This can give one something of a jolt. However, many more women are having babies later in life, and I know that in my antenatal clinic women find considerable comfort in meeting others who thought they were much too old to cope with pregnancy.

Some older women do feel more tired than their younger counterparts both during pregnancy and after it. Nearly all pregnant women get fatigued, and those who are older than average may need a bit more rest than usual. Very many women in this situation lose confidence in themselves and feel full of doubt. I feel that one can be truly fortunate to be pregnant at forty and privileged to be in a position of very special fulfilment and enjoyment.

Being older also has one other great advantage – being more experienced in life and more mature. Older women can often be a bit more assertive than younger mothers in the average antenatal clinic. People should not be afraid of being persistent until they get clear explanations from their doctor and midwives about what they have in mind. Older mothers generally will find it much easier to get information than many younger women. Being as old as (or even older than) some of the doctors and nurses can be a very great advantage.

Modern reproductive technology and older women

In the last two years or so there has been growing interest in more active treatment of infertile women, using advanced methods such as test-tube baby treatment (IVF), or egg donation.

IVF AND OLDER WOMEN

As we shall see in Chapter 11, IVF frequently involves the transfer of more than one embryo to the uterus. In very good IVF units, where the chance of each embryo implanting is comparatively high, transfer of more than one embryo simultaneously can result in higher than natural chances of conception, when normally only one egg is ovulated.

EGG DONATION

As we have seen, the most important reason why older women fail to conceive is because their eggs are abnormal. One way around this problem is to use donor eggs from younger women. They can be fertilised with the older woman's husband's sperm, and then transferred to the older woman's uterus. It does not matter if the woman has reached the menopause, and stopped menstruating. Drugs (a strong form of hormone replacement therapy) are given to encourage regular periods for two months, a younger woman's ovaries are stimulated with fertility injection and the egg collected surgically, and any resulting embryos may be given to the older woman at the correct time in her medically induced menstrual cycle.

This treatment has been used in New York, and to some extent in England. In some units, treatment with donor eggs has been put to extremes. In Rome, where it seems there are people who are prepared to pay for anything, a fertility doctor called Dr Antinori has been using donated eggs from young women and has transferred them to the uterus of women in their late fifties, or even early sixties – well after the menopause. A recent BBC television programme *The Heart of the Matter* highlighted his work. He claimed that he saw nothing wrong or alarming in this and seemed surprised that doctors in Britain were concerned. My own feeling is that it is very unwise to treat most women much beyond their late forties in this way for a number of cogent reasons:

1. The risks of serious medical disorders of pregnancy, such as high blood pressure, diabetes and heart disease, do grow significantly in women over fifty.

2. The higher risk of miscarriage means that a desperate woman may be badly emotionally damaged by losing a pregnancy at the very end of reproductive life.

3. The use of donated eggs takes no account of the donor who may imagine that her eggs are going to help a woman of her own age and therefore someone whom she may feel is more suitable to look after a baby.

4. Donor eggs are in very short supply and probably better reserved for women who are infertile as a result of diseases such as premature menopause, rather than for women who are trying to buck a natural biological event (e.g., the menopause).

5. Most importantly, it takes no account of any resulting child whose mother will be well over sixty years old (if still alive), before he or she is a teenager.

Whilst I have every sympathy for older menopausal women who wish to conceive, I feel that egg donation is a step too far in most cases. I do not think egg donation is generally a suitable treatment for women who are simply 'too old to have a child'.

PART TWO

IF PREGNANCY DOESN'T HAPPEN

CHAPTER SIX

The Causes of Female Infertility

We humans are among the least fertile members of the animal kingdom. Even totally healthy women do not ovulate each menstrual cycle. Moreover, blocked Fallopian tubes or abnormalities of the uterus are probably much more common in women than in animal species. And to make matters worse, the human male tends to produce more abnormal sperm.

In the past, it was widely supposed that infertility was a female 'fault', and this belief resulted in a totally unreasonable burden being placed on many childless women. This depressingly chauvinistic attitude is still prevalent in some primitive societies and regrettably, even in developed countries an irrational 'female' stigma is widely attached to infertility. However, two things are clear. One is that infertility is rarely any person's 'fault'. Men and women, and particularly the latter, often believe that they are infertile because, in the past, they have done something that has led to the problem. However, as we shall see, this is seldom true. The other thing that should be understood is that infertility is just as likely to be the man's problem as it is to be the woman's. Statistics show that, in Europe, only in about one-third of cases is the cause of infertility due to some failure of the woman's reproductive function; in another third, the man will be solely responsible. In the cases remaining, both partners contribute to the problem in some degree.

Few couples are worried if they do not conceive within a few months of trying. The gradual realisation that there may be something wrong is often not talked about, but underneath people feel increasing anxiety. Usually, the woman takes the initiative by going to see the doctor, sometimes when her partner is not fully aware of her worries. Matters may come to a head when a couple find friends and relatives starting families without difficulty; and as they become increasingly aware that they have a problem, they frequently experience anger, frustration and, commonly, a loss of self-esteem. Persistent infertility can be very corrosive, and readers who have found themselves in this situation may well feel very sad and tearful. In particular, the grief of infertility often makes people feel guilty, as if they have actually caused their own problem. I have found that, if a man and a woman can find the reason for their infertility, it is very much easier to come to terms with the distress it causes – and it makes any treatment to overcome it much more likely to succeed.

Failure to ovulate

The most common reason why a woman may not be able to conceive is a failure to ovulate. This accounts for about 30 per cent of female infertility. Fortunately, this is usually treatable by the use of fertility drugs (*see* Chapter 9). Why so many women fail to ovulate is not understood completely, but we know a number of reasons for it.

HORMONAL PROBLEMS

Sometimes there is a problem with the hormones secreted by the ovaries themselves, by the hypothalamus in the brain, by the pituitary gland at the base of the brain, or by the thyroid gland in the neck.

● *Failure to produce mature eggs.* In about half the cases of failure to ovulate, the ovaries do not regularly produce properly mature follicles in which the eggs can adequately develop. If they are not fully mature, it is unlikely that ovulation will occur, but even if it does, the eggs may fail to become fertilised. The most common disorder responsible for this is *polycystic ovary syndrome*, which may be caused by an imbalance between the hormones of the ovaries and those of the adrenal glands (just above the kidneys), or by an abnormality of the hypothalamus (*see* below).

● *Malfunction of the hypothalamus.* This is the part of the brain that sends signals to the pituitary gland, which in turn sends hormonal messages to the ovaries to cause them to produce mature eggs. In about 20 per cent of ovulation failure, malfunction of the hypothalamus is the basic cause.

● *Malfunction of the pituitary gland.* If the pituitary does not produce enough – or if it produces too much – of the ovary-stimulating hormones, the ovaries will be incapable of proper ovulation. This can happen if there is a chemical imbalance in the pituitary, or if it is physically injured.

● *Thyroid problems.* These are relatively rare, and require blood tests to identify them.

WHAT TO LOOK OUT FOR

● Infrequent periods, occurring at longer than thirty-six-day intervals. Occasionally there are no periods at all. Often periods may be very scanty, with hardly any bleeding. However, some women who are not ovulating may have normal periods.

● Weight gain. Excess body fat is definitely often associated with a failure to ovulate.[16] Those who think this may be the problem would be well advised to go on a sensible diet. This should not be overdone – losing too much weight can also cause infertility problems.

● Excessive exercise. There is now good evidence that repeated, vigorous exercise stops some women from ovulating. For example, running long distances every day may be harmful.

---

[16] I find this extremely hard to get across to my overweight infertile patients, who often recall that fatness is frequently associated with having large numbers of babies. That may be true, but fat women – when they do have ovulatory problems – are much more difficult to treat successfully, and run greater risks from the results of treatment.

If the periods are irregular, it may be well to cut down on physical training.

● New excessive body and/or facial hair. This is often a sign of polycystic ovaries.

SCARRED OVARIES

Physical damage to the ovaries can undoubtedly cause failure to ovulate. Sometimes the capsule of the ovary (its outer skin) can become so scarred after extensive, repeated surgery (perhaps for ovarian cysts), particularly if this is also associated with infection so that the follicles cannot develop properly. This can be a side-effect of pelvic radiation therapy for cancer.

WHAT TO LOOK FOR

There is usually a medical history of multiple pelvic infections or repeated pelvic surgery, sometimes for the removal of cysts from one or both ovaries.

PREMATURE MENOPAUSE

A somewhat uncommon cause of ovulatory failure is premature menopause, or premature ovarian failure. Some women, for reasons that are not well understood, seem to run out of eggs well before the usual age for the 'change of life', and the level of the female hormone oestrogen in their blood is comparatively low. Menstruation stops completely, and menopausal symptoms such as hot flushes and dry vagina are common. The resulting infertility is usually not directly treatable, although hormone replacement therapy (HRT) will control the symptoms of premature menopause completely. Recently, however, childbearing has been made possible through in vitro fertilisation by using eggs from a donor (see p. 94).

Premature menopause may be genetic. The condition certainly seems to run in families. In addition, there are certain genetic abnormalities that can result in girls being born with little or no ovarian tissue – *ovarian agenesis*. The most common is Turner's syndrome, caused by the absence of one of the female X-chromosomes. Those who have this condition are usually shorter than average, and frequently have other problems as well, so that Turner's syndrome is almost always diagnosed before puberty. On rare occasions, premature menopause may also be due to an immune phenomenon. The precise mechanism is not understood, but it seems that the body can manufacture antibodies which attack ovarian tissue, causing complete ovarian failure.

WHAT TO LOOK FOR

● Complete loss of periods or bleeding only at very infrequent intervals.
● Hot flushes and/or dry vagina.

It is important to recognise, however, that these are very common symptoms and may not mean that a woman is not producing eggs.

FOLLICLE PROBLEMS

Some women appear to produce at monthly intervals a good follicle in which an egg develops, but for unknown reasons the follicle does not rupture on time and therefore the egg remains trapped inside the ovary. The mechanism behind this 'unruptured follicle syndrome' is poorly understood, but it is receiving great attention from doctors in various parts of the world.

PSYCHOLOGICAL REASONS

Most women, at some time during their lives, have a month or two when they do not ovulate. This most commonly occurs when they come under severe stress: during exams, after the loss of a job or the death of someone close to them, during and after marital break-up, because of a bout of very bad depression. However, some women temporarily lose their ability to ovulate after far less traumatic emotional events.

Continued stress is only very rarely a cause of persistent failure to ovulate, and it is most unlikely that much infertility is caused by psychological disturbance.

WHAT TO LOOK OUT FOR

Menstrual delay or irregularity are likely particularly when under stress.

Damaged Fallopian tubes

Fortunately, tubal damage seldom harms a woman's general health, and because of this, doctors believe that there is hardly ever any justification for treatment unless pregnancy is desired. As we shall see later, the most effective form of treatment is tubal microsurgery.

INFLAMMATION ASSOCIATED WITH INFECTION

Different micro-organisms – bacteria, viruses and others – can cause tubal scarring and other damage. It is often thought that tubal infection – or *salpingitis*, to give it its proper medical name – is always the result of promiscuity leading to sexually transmitted disease (formerly called venereal disease). This is, however, definitely untrue. Although salpingitis is rare in virgins and is more common in women who have regular sexual intercourse, it can be caused by many micro-organisms that are naturally found in the body, including *E.coli*, found in the bowel, and various forms of *Streptococci*, often in the vagina of perfectly fertile women.

However, the sexual pathway cannot be completely ruled

out. Gonorrhoea is a major transmitted disease that can cause salpingitis, and chlamydia, micro-organisms halfway between bacteria and viruses, accounting for perhaps 15 per cent of all tubal damage, may be transmitted by sexual contact.

Those women who are unfortunate enough to have tubal damage, possibly caused by an infection, are likely to ask how the infection was 'caught' and whether their partner was responsible. Many of my patients finally bring themselves to ask me whether I think that they have caught a tubal infection from their husband or a boyfriend. The answer is almost invariably 'No'. Detailed research at our clinic a few years ago showed that perhaps no more than 10 per cent of women with tubal damage had definitely had a sexually transmitted infection.

INFLAMMATION ASSOCIATED WITH ABDOMINAL DISEASE

The most important of these diseases is appendicitis, especially if there is also peritonitis (a generalised infection of the abdominal cavity caused, in this case, by a burst appendix), but some forms of colitis (a bowel condition) may also be responsible. Inflammation of the abdominal cavity or the bowel can spread to involve the Fallopian tubes, which subsequently become scarred and blocked. Fortunately, although appendicitis is very common, it only rarely results in the tubes being damaged.

INFLAMMATION FOLLOWING CHILDBIRTH, MISCARRIAGE OR ABORTION

The uterus and the tubes are particularly susceptible to infection immediately after pregnancy. This is slightly more likely if delivery of a baby has been complicated – for example, if it has been a forceps delivery. After miscarriage, it is more apt to occur if an operation had been needed to remove all the tissue.

In the past – and today in countries where therapeutic abortions are illegal – back-street, hastily conducted illegal terminations of pregnancy led very frequently to serious infertility afterwards. This is now rare in most developed countries, largely because abortions can be performed without any serious health risk. Nevertheless, it is extremely common for infertile women to wonder whether it is because they once had a termination that they are infertile now.

It is hardly surprising that people who are in this situation may well feel that they have brought this all on themselves, no matter how irrational this belief may be. Guilt about the past is quite a common emotion, but things should be kept in perspective. The vast majority of the hundreds of thousands of women who have abortions every year have decided that this was the best course of action for them at a very difficult time. A past abortion only rarely causes a present problem; for example, some infection which left the uterus or tubes scarred. This is generally uncommon. Couples should try to draw a firm line across this past and look positively at what is occurring now. If this proves difficult, counselling can be extremely helpful.

SURGICAL DAMAGE

A most important cause of tubal disease and subsequent damage is previous abdominal or pelvic surgery, particularly an operation on the uterus, Fallopian tubes or ovaries. Such operations, if they are done without a microscope (i.e. using conventional rather than microsurgical techniques), can lead to adhesions that may 'glue' the tubes down so that eggs cannot travel through them.

ECTOPIC PREGNANCY

A pregnancy that occurs in one or other tube (see Chapter 13) often leads to scarring, which can cause tubal damage. Conversely and more importantly, tubal damage can lead to ectopic pregnancy.

CONGENITAL DEFECT

A few women are born with an abnormality of one or both tubes. This may also be associated with abnormalities of the uterus (*see* below).

ENDOMETRIOSIS

Endometriosis is a condition where the lining of the uterus, the endometrium, grows not only inside the uterus but also in the abdomen. Occasionally, it can lead to severe scarring of the tubes or adhesions.

WHAT TO LOOK FOR

In most cases, women with tubal damage are completely free of any symptoms. However, there may be:
● quite severe period pains, or pain on intercourse;
● a history of pelvic infection, cystitis-like episodes that were never properly diagnosed, or a burst appendix.

An abnormal uterus

Problems in the womb itself account for at least 10 per cent of all cases of female infertility, but despite this, testing to see if the uterus or its cavity are abnormal is often not done. This is a source of amazement to me – after all, the sperm have to pass through the uterus on their way to fertilise the egg, and the developing baby implants and grows there.

FIBROIDS

These are very common, benign (non-cancerous) tumours that can grow in almost any part of the uterus. Many women who have them are completely fertile, and it may be that infertility occurs only when they grow in particular places – in the uterine cavity, or so that they block the Fallopian tubes or dislodge the ovaries from their normal position.

Why they grow at all is a total mystery. We do know that they are much more common in women over the age of thirty-five and that they do not develop after the menopause. There also seems to be a genetic predisposition to fibroids – they often affect more than one female member of a family, and certain racial groups, such as black African women, are more prone to them. However, fibroids are so common that about 1 in every 3 women will have some by the age of forty. This may sound a little frightening, but it is rare for fibroids to cause any serious problems – apart from infertility.

WHAT TO LOOK OUT FOR

- Increasingly heavy and painful periods.
- Swelling in the abdomen.

Many other conditions can also cause these very common symptoms, but infertility may be the only sign that something is wrong.

ADENOMYOSIS

This condition is perhaps rather more common than is often thought. Normally the lining of the uterus – the endometrium – is shed each month at menstruation. However, in adenomyosis, some lining grows into the thick muscle of the uterus and, consequently, menstrual bleeding occurs there. Usually only isolated areas are affected, but occasionally the whole of the uterine muscle wall is involved. The uterine lining can also grow into a Fallopian tube near the junction with the uterus, which can cause scarring and block the tube partially or completely.

WHAT TO LOOK OUT FOR

● Prolonged, painful periods; often the pain is dull and continuous.
● Occasionally the uterus may be enlarged and a bit tender.
● Dull pain on intercourse.

CONGENITAL ABNORMALITIES

A surprising number of perfectly healthy women are born with an abnormality of the uterus. In many cases, this does not cause infertility, and they may go through life without knowing that their uteruses are any different from anybody else's.

In all mammals – rabbits, cats, dogs, sheep, whales, monkeys, humans – the uterus develops from two separate tubes in the abdomen of the embryo, one on the right side of the body and the other on the left. In monkeys and humans, these two tubes become fused together to form one cavity with one womb. However, virtually all other mammals develop two separate uteruses on either side of the abdomen.

Because the human uterus grows from the two tubes fusing together, most abnormalities result from incomplete fusion. In some cases, the embryonic tubes fail to stick together at all, resulting in the woman having two uteruses, both smaller than one fused uterus. This may cause infertility and, not infrequently, recurrent miscarriages. Much more common, however, is a *septate uterus* – a protrusion into the upper part of the uterine cavity. This may cause no problems, but it is known to be associated with miscarriage, rather than an inability to conceive.

As well as problems with conception and miscarriage, these abnormalities can sometimes cause unusually painful periods. They may also lead to problems during childbirth, for example,

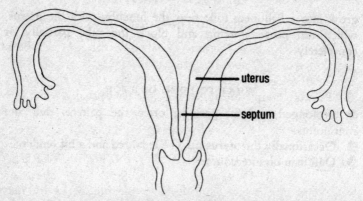

A septate uterus, a common cause of both infertility and miscarriages. Although the inside of the uterus is very indented by the septum, note that outside it has a normal contour. A septate uterus may therefore not be apparent on laparoscopy alone, and X-ray is usually essential.

the baby may lie in the breech position, or there may be trouble delivering the placenta at the end of labour.

UTERINE ADHESIONS

About half the women with uterine problems that we see have adhesions in the inside of the uterus. This means that the internal walls of the uterus are stuck together, causing the cavity to be distorted. The problem usually follows a previous pregnancy.

This condition is frequently referred to as *Asherman's syndrome*, after Dr Asherman of Jerusalem who first described it in 1947. He felt that these adhesions nearly always followed physical trauma, usually injury to the walls of the uterus following a curettage ('scrape' or D & C) after a miscarriage or termination of pregnancy.

WHAT TO LOOK OUT FOR

● Periods that have become scanty or stop altogether following a miscarriage, abortion, difficult delivery or removal of a uterine fibroid.

● Painful cramps during periods, the pain usually when flow is heaviest.

POLYPS OR FOREIGN BODY IN THE UTERUS

Any solid object that obtrudes into the uterine cavity may prevent a pregnancy. Indeed, this is how the contraceptive coil (IUD) works.

Solid uterine objects are not that common. They include polyps – fleshy, grape-like growths of the uterine lining that are not shed – and small fibroids. Very occasionally, there may be a forgotten contraceptive coil, or part of one if it has been incompletely removed.

WHAT TO LOOK OUT FOR

There are often no symptoms. However, there may be painful cramps during periods, sometimes heavy bleeding, and occasionally, spotting between periods.

Problems with the cervix

The cervix performs two vital functions in conception and pregnancy. First, it acts as an important reservoir for sperm. After sex, the sperm stay in the cervical mucus, from where they swim up into the uterus and through into the Fallopian tubes to meet the egg.

Second, the cervix holds the uterus shut once pregnancy occurs so that the developing embryo and foetus are kept safely inside to develop completely.

PROBLEMS WITH THE CERVICAL MUCUS

There are several reasons why sperm may not survive in the cervical mucus. It may not be of good quality because hormone levels are wrong. Adequate amounts of watery mucus in which the sperm can swim easily are made in the cervix in response to the hormone oestrogen. Virtually the only time during the menstrual cycle when conditions are right for sperm is just before ovulation (this is why checking the condition of cervical mucus is used in some forms of birth control). Thick mucus, on the other hand, is made in response to the hormone *progesterone*, which is usually produced *after* ovulation. If the body is not producing enough oestrogen, the mucus may be scanty or very thick and the sperm may not be able to swim through it to reach the egg. The most common reason why insufficient oestrogen is produced is failure of ovulation (*see* p. 100).

There may be various reasons why the secreting cells of the cervix cannot make enough good mucus. The causes and treatment of cervical problems are described on pp. 268 and 275.

PROBLEMS WITH AN OPEN CERVIX

If the membrances surrounding the developing baby 'pout' through the opening of a cervix that is abnormally widened, infection can set in, the membranes can rupture and miscarriage or early labour occurs. This disaster is, unfortunately, quite common. A miscarriage between sixteen to twenty-six weeks after conception indicates that possibly the cervix opened, suggesting what is referred to as an *incompetent cervix*. It may occur because of a congenital weakness in the muscles of the cervix or follow injury – for example, if the cervix has been damaged during an operation to remove the remaining products of conception following a miscarriage, or during a complicated delivery or late abortion. Luckily, in the great majority of cases, this condition is easy to treat with a stitch to keep the cervix shut.

CHAPTER SEVEN

The Causes of Male Infertility

At least 30 per cent of infertility is due to a problem in the man. In spite of this, it is surprising how often the burden of infertility is borne by female partners. Most infertility specialists, for example, are gynaecologists – that is specialists in the medicine and surgery of the female reproductive system. Indeed, in Britain at least, there are very few *andrologists* (specialists in the male reproductive system). In many infertility clinics, the woman is often seen by herself and she alone is examined. The male is relegated to merely providing a sperm specimen. This traditional view of infertility is outmoded and wrong. In my view, wherever possible a couple should go together to a specialist if they are seeking help.

Unfortunately, male infertility carries a stigma. Consequently, very many men are reluctant to have tests. When a woman is infertile, she quite often has some physical symptoms; she may therefore go to her doctor with some idea that her body isn't working normally. Male infertility seldom causes symptoms, and this is one reason why some men resist becoming involved with tests. This refusal can cause friction between a man and a woman, especially if there is a likelihood of there being a male problem.

Many men are more distressed at being infertile than their partners. Some become very disturbed, or clinically depressed. Finding that their sperm count is low means that they are responsible, the guilty one. They live with a sense of loss and can, quite illogically, feel deeply ashamed. Male infertility, by its very nature, usually hits a man between the ages of twenty-five and forty-five, when he may be trying to establish himself in other ways, perhaps in a better job. Frequently the sense of failure spills over into other aspects of his life, such as failed professional ambitions.

Of course, a woman may be upset about her partner's infertility, but generally the extent of these feelings seems greater to her partner than they really are. She may indeed feel angry at being denied a child through no fault of her own, but this anger conflicts with her love and feeling for her partner so that she becomes very confused. Most women patients I know would much prefer the problem to be theirs; they feel that they would find it easier to deal with emotionally, fearing the effect that the diagnosis of subfertility or infertility will have on their partners. Often they resist that their men be tested and try to shelter them. They may go through all sorts of tests without even telling their partners that they are attending an infertility clinic. Other women find that their partners will not see a doctor, nor will they produce sperm for testing. These men neither want the ordeal of the test nor admit why they feel it is an adverse reflection on their sexuality.

It is quite common for people to think that they are inadequate sexually simply because they can't have children. Men feel this particularly. There is widespread confusion between infertility and sexual performance, virility and masculinity. In fact, there is no connection and a man's potency is in no way related to his ability to produce sperm. Equally, men who are impotent and unable to give their partners any pleasure at all through sexual intercourse are as likely as the rest of the population to be perfectly fertile.

These sexual feelings may present themselves in different ways in the doctor's consulting room. Sheila and Joseph, a very happily married couple, originally consulted us because they had been trying to get pregnant for seven years; before they were seen by us they had been told that there was no explanation for their infertility. Testing in our clinic clearly showed that there was a real reason for the problem, namely that Joseph was mostly producing very abnormal sperm which were quite incapable of fertilising eggs. Only a few of the sperm were normal, just sufficient for them to be considered for test-tube baby treatment (IVF). They were placed on the waiting list for this to be done, which at that time was about ten months long. Four months later, they came back to see me and asked for Sheila to have artificial insemination with Joseph's semen until the time came for IVF. I pointed out that insemination would be unlikely to help and that natural intercourse was much more successful. At this point, Sheila burst into tears. It gradually came out that, since we had firmly established the cause of the infertility, Joseph had become completely impotent. It took a good deal of treatment and counselling before these sexual difficulties were resolved.

Why are some men infertile?

NO SPERM IN THE SEMEN FLUID

Occasionally no sperm are being produced in the semen. This may be because none is being made by the testicle, or because they are not being ejaculated during orgasm. Failure to ejaculate sperm in spite of their production by the testicle is due either to the tubes from the testicles to the seminal vesicles being blocked (see illustration on p. 19), or to the muscles that pump semen through the urethra not working properly.

It is rare for the testicles to fail to make any sperm at all. Fewer than 5 per cent of infertile men have this problem. Just as complete ovarian failure in women is usually untreatable, total failure of the testicle is very difficult to alter. Usually it is impossible to find the cause. It may be due to a hard blow to the testicles, such as a sporting injury, a previous severe mumps infection, or damage to the blood supply to the testicle, usually due to a serious twisting of the testicles. If this is the case, the doctor may make the diagnosis easily from discussing the man's past medical history.

Testicular failure may also have a hormonal cause. The

pituitary gland in the brain may not produce enough hormones to stimulate the testicles. Alternatively, the testicles may not respond to these hormones for several, mostly uncommon, reasons:

● The man's testicles did not descend into the scrotum after birth and they are usually not properly developed and cannot make sperm.

● The cells of the testicles are unable to make sperm even when there is enough male hormone.

● There is a rare defect from birth. This is likely to be chromosomal.

These three conditions are usually untreatable, although in rare cases, hormones may help.

● If the minute tubes that connect the testicles to the seminal vesicles are blocked, the testicles may produce sperm but these cannot get into the semen. Blockage of these tubes is a result of scarring, often due to an infection such as gonorrhoea or tuberculosis, occasionally because of injury and sometimes as a birth defect. Such blocks may be amenable to surgery.

In about 1 per cent of cases, the genital muscles do not pump in a properly coordinated way during orgasm. Sperm may enter the bladder and mix with the urine, rather than get into the woman's vagina. This is called *retrograde ejaculation* and may follow an operation such as the removal of the prostate gland. It may also happen if the nerves to the muscles are damaged. Some drugs, particularly tranquillisers and those used to control high blood pressure, may also temporarily cause this.

THE SEMEN CONTAINS FEW SPERM

The vast majority of cases of male infertility (about 70 per cent) are due to a low sperm count. There are very many reasons for this, but most of the time the real cause cannot be established with any certainty. Regrettably, when the count is low, many of the sperm which are present in the semen are frequently either of poor motility (i.e. they do not move properly) or they are abnormal in some way (*see* below).

If the sperm count is low but the sperm themselves are quite normal, the outlook is good. Most men in this situation are very likely to get their partner pregnant eventually, though often it may take very much longer than normal for this happy outcome.

SPERM THAT ARE LARGELY ABNORMAL OR OF LOW MOTILITY

There are many reasons why sperm is abnormal, but in most cases a definite cause cannot be found. In many men, there is probably a genetic defect which accounts for this. Also, as a man gets older more of his sperm tend to be abnormal or of low motility. Some of the known causes include:

● *Hormonal problems* which may drastically reduce sperm quality. Generally, the more severe the hormonal problem, the worse will be the sperm motility or quality.

● *Abnormal blood vessels around the testicle* may be associated with 'bad' sperm. There may be enlarged veins, rather like varicose veins, draining the testicles. This condition is known as *varicocoele* and is thought by some people to cause overheating of the testicles. Varicocoeles are usually quite painless and seldom even tender. They do not interfere with sex unless knocked very hard indeed in a moment of great passion. The blood in the enlarged veins may indeed be keeping it at a higher temperature than normal, but this is almost certainly not the whole story (remember the elephant in Chapter 1?). The real reason why a varicocoele causes some men to be infertile but not others is not yet known.

● *An infection* that has lasted a long time is sometimes thought to cause poor sperm quality. An infection of the prostate gland may be found in a few men with poor sperm. Some doctors believe that one group of microbes – the *mycoplasmas* – are particularly likely to cause problems, perhaps by reducing sperm motility. The mycoplasmas have recently come under considerable scientific scrutiny. There is good evidence in animals that these organisms may interfere with the ability of sperm to fertilise an egg. Although these microbes are not at all dangerous to general health, antibiotics may be given in an attempt to improve the quality of the sperm.

Sometimes sperm that look normal under the microscope are actually chemically abnormal. This is not common, but is seldom treatable with drugs.

IMMUNOLOGICAL PROBLEMS

About 5 per cent of male infertility is caused by an immune reaction. For reasons that are not yet known, some men form antibodies to their own sperm. The body 'sees' the sperm as 'foreign' and attacks them with its immune defences. This action is very similar to how the body protects itself from being invaded by foreign proteins, bacteria or cells. Unfortunately, in this situation it causes an unwanted consequence. Why antibodies occur is uncertain, but they may be a response to some kind of injury earlier in life.

DIFFICULTY WITH INTERCOURSE

Difficulty with sexual intercourse is very rarely the cause of male infertility (less than 1 per cent). Sexual difficulties can result in sperm not being ejaculated into the vagina. The commonest problem is what is called *premature ejaculation*, when the man has his orgasm before he is able to get the penis deep into the vagina. This is more likely in very young men and can be overcome with patience and practice.

There are many other reasons for difficulty with intercourse, and these are outside the scope of this book. Sexual problems need specialised help, and the best people to consult are often counsellors trained in marriage guidance. Family doctors can suggest the best sources of help. Although many men may, at first, feel too embarrassed to discuss this, sympathetic advice is readily available from those familiar with these problems.

ANATOMICAL ABNORMALITIES

These are also very rare. The most common is the condition known as *hypospadias*, when the urethra (the tube running through the penis) opens into the outside world underneath the penis or even near the scrotum. As with retrograde ejaculation, sperm are not ejaculated into the vagina. This can be treated with a simple operation.

Absence of the vas deferens, or poorly developed testicles are other rare anatomical abnormalities that can affect fertility.

ENVIRONMENTAL FACTORS

Certain environmental factors contribute to reduced sperm production and poor sperm quality. Severe pressure of work, smoking and excessive alcohol all can result in a reduction of male fertility. This is very important as often these factors are very easily corrected (*see* pp. 157–8). There are a number of reasons why a man's sperm count can be depressed.

● *Smoking*. This may have no effect on many men with completely normal or high sperm counts. However, if a man is prone to under-produce sperm, he may have a catastrophic drop in sperm numbers and quality if he smokes.

● *Alcohol*. Like tobacco, alcohol is a poison, and it damages the cells which make sperm. In most men, heavy drinking over a period of time is likely to reduce their ability to make sperm. Different men have a different tolerance to alcohol, but it is certainly important for a man to restrict his drinking if he is prone to this problem.

● *Excessive exercise*. Regular sport, jogging or cycling promotes well-being, but there is evidence that excessive strenuous exercise may affect sperm production.[17] We know that some

---

[17] Many years ago an England cricketer consulted me about persistent infertility. Thorough examination failed to reveal anything wrong with either his wife or himself, although sperm tests were a bit low. Careful history-taking showed that his international schedule precluded his having a normal marital

athletes at the peak of training have reduced sperm counts, but these return to normal when they exercise less and gain a little weight.

● *Being overweight.* Although many obese men are fertile, there is an increased chance of infertility if a man is overweight.

● *Caffeine.* There is increasing evidence that both excessive coffee and tea drinking may be associated with both male and female infertility. In men, this is caused by sperm defects; the reason why it prevents women conceiving is not understood.

● *Drugs.* Some drugs reduce sperm count. On the list of 'social' drugs is cannabis (marijuana) which can have a powerful effect on the sperm of some men. There are a number of medicinal drugs that may depress sperm count and the doctor should be asked about this if medication is being taken for any reason.

● *Frequent sex.* Some people think the quality and quantity of their sperm may be reduced if they have sex too often. This has not been proved, and I don't believe it. Having said that, sport can have other effects. I once treated a couple from Tottenham – nothing could be found beyond a rather poor sperm count. I asked the wife, who looked wan and tired, how often they had sex and she told me, with no particular emotion, that she and her husband had made love six times every night for the last five years. Apparently, they had never missed an evening except two nights while the Football World Cup was televised. With great difficulty, I tried to persuade them that this might be a little over-indulgent. She eventually conceived the week Spurs won the FA Cup Final, in 1991.

● *The stresses of work and daily life.* This is a most difficult factor to weigh up. It is always a problem to understand just which aspects of anyone's life may be contributing to poor fertility. At particular risk are people such as the high-powered executive, who is constantly flying around the world and is

existence; at that time England team managers refused to allow wives or girlfriends to go on tour, severely limiting when he spent so much time in Australia, South Africa and India. Happily, after a bad season with the bat, he lost his England cap and promptly gained two children in rapid succession.

under pressure all the time. To make matters worse, he may often be away from home for long periods, perhaps at those times when his wife is most fertile. Apart from reducing the chance of conception, time away from home throws added strain on the sexual and marital relationship, compounding stress. These professional pressures are often worst when a man is in his thirties and early forties, yet this may be the best time to have a child, particularly as a woman's fertility is decreasing as time creeps on. High rates of stress are also experienced by those in low-skill manual jobs, such as assembly workers.

● *Occupational hazards*. Other occupations associated with sperm problems include those involving long-distance driving or jobs where there is exposure to poisonous substances such as lead – for example, lead-laden petrol fumes in a bus depot. Men exposed to excessive vibration, such as boiler-makers or pneumatic drill operators, or those in any other job where the environment is very tiring or stressful, may also be affected.

CHAPTER EIGHT

Investigating Infertility

When to test for infertility

It is not worth worrying unless there has been no conception after regular sex without contraception for six months at least. In couples where the woman is under thirty, it is reasonable to wait two years before tests. If the woman is over thirty, there is a bit more urgency. At this age, people naturally feel that time is running out. Here is a paradox: as the older woman tends to be a little less fertile anyway, she may naturally take longer to conceive. Nevertheless, I recommend comprehensive tests to anyone in this age group.

Some people may want earlier investigation than I have recommended. This may be because there is a good reason to believe that there is a definite problem. With any of the following symptoms, it might be silly to wait too long before tests are done:

HISTORY/SYMPTOMS	POSSIBLE CAUSE/RESULT
WOMAN	
No periods for some time	Probably not ovulating
Very infrequent periods	Not ovulating regularly
Painful periods *and* deep pain on sex	Inflammation or endometriosis
Recent very heavy periods	Problem in the uterus
Previous operation for ovarian cyst	Adhesions

Previous burst appendix	Tubal problems
History of infection with contraceptive coil	Adhesions
Previous infection immediately after pregnancy	Pelvic inflammation

MAN

Mumps during adult life	Poor sperm production
Definite testicle injury	Poor sperm production
Undescended testicle	Poor/absent sperms

This list is not exhaustive, but it does contain the more common reasons for seeking early help. People who think they may have another problem should certainly consult their family doctor, who will be able to offer advice.

FIRST FIND THE CAUSE

This is the single, most important piece of advice in this book. It is crucial to understand that infertility itself is not a disease. It is a symptom that something is not quite right with one or even both partners. Before having treatment for infertility, it is essential that proper tests are carried out to find the cause. If this is not done, the wrong treatment may be given, with inevitable delays in solving the problem. For example, far too many women are given fertility pills when they first go to their doctor complaining of difficulty in conceiving. This is a mistake. First, not only might it delay finding the real cause of their trouble, which results in a delay in their getting effective treatment for the real cause, but inappropriate treatment may prevent conception. For example, clomiphene tablets (brand name Clomid, the most common fertility pill) can actually prevent women conceiving if they do not have a problem with ovulation.

To take another example, sometimes people think that if they just ask for IVF, they will be successful. This is like the man who goes to his GP with pain in the chest, and asks for radiotherapy. He may have bronchitis, in which case he needs an antibiotic; perhaps he has indigestion, in which case an antacid; possibly a broken rib, in which case some strapping; or maybe heart disease, in which case he needs more tests. The chance he has lung cancer, in which case he really needs radiotherapy, is unlikely.

TRYING TO ENSURE REASONABLY PROMPT DIAGNOSIS

Once the decision to have infertility tests has been taken, a diagnosis should usually be made well within six months. A few couples, especially younger ones, may decide to have a few simple tests and then await events. Generally, though, once tests have started, it is probably best to establish the cause (or causes) of the problem so that one knows where one stands. One of the most common failures in the treatment of infertility is to allow the tests to drift on, often for years. This may result in a couple receiving inadequate or wrong treatment simply because the cause has not been correctly established. This can have tragic consequences, especially if the woman is in her late thirties and time is running out. A common problem is when one cause is found halfway through infertility testing and treatment is immediately started without completing other tests. A couple may well have more than one problem contributing to their failure to conceive, and treatment of one without discovering the other will prolong things unnecessarily.

Even experienced specialists (myself very much included) may occasionally forget to perform an important test. Although people may be in awe of their specialist (a totally illogical attitude in my view), the specialist should certainly be reminded if the patient feels that a particular test might be helpful. This chapter provides you with a checklist. Many patients find it very difficult or embarrassing to be assertive. Those who cannot summon up the courage to ask the specialist should talk things over with their family doctor. After all, he or she will have usually made the original referral to the specialist. The family doctor is there, above all, to keep a watching brief over one's general care. People should feel free to tell their family doctor that certain tests are taking too long, or are not being done. A letter from him or her to the specialist, outlining these concerns, will frequently speed things up dramatically. The specialist will seldom take offence. On the contrary, the specialist's practice depends on him or her satisfying the patients sent by family doctors.

WHAT TESTS MAY BE HELPFUL BEFORE SEEKING SPECIALIST HELP?

In the early days of trying for a baby, three simple tests may help identify a problem. These can be organised by family doctors before referral to a specialist is considered.

● *Temperature charting*. A woman's temperature rises slightly after ovulation and remains raised until the next menstrual period. A woman should consider taking her temperature for two or three months to see if there is evidence of ovulating. Unfortunately, this test is not 100 per cent reliable, but may be an indicator.

● *The woman can have a blood test* to see if she is ovulating. The family doctor can easily arrange to have blood progesterone levels measured in the second half of the menstrual cycle. A well-raised level is excellent evidence of ovulation.

● *The man could have a simple sperm test*. This may show that there are inadequate numbers of normal sperm, in which case early specialist referral is justified.

REFERRAL TO A SPECIALIST OR INFERTILITY CLINIC

If after two years conception has not happened, or if one is in any of the situations I have already described, the family doctor will suggest referral to a specialist. This will usually be a consultant, often a gynaecologist, who has an interest in infertility. Those people who have a clinic or specialist in mind and who would like to be specifically referred there, should remember that they are entitled to ask this of their family doctor. Many people worry about whether the woman should go on her own, or whether both partners should go to the specialist for the first visit. Generally, I think it is better if the couple attends together – for the first appointment, at least – as this means that the tensions involved in clinic visits in a possibly forbidding hospital can be shared. Most specialists are pleased if both partners come.

What happens at a first appointment?

In the previous chapters, we looked at various symptoms. These lead to the main questions one might expect the doctor to ask. Obviously, age is important and the length of time a couple have been trying to have a baby. A history of any previous pregnancies is important and whether the woman found it difficult to conceive them. If the woman used to get pregnant easily, it suggests that something has happened to change her fertility.

Some woman are very worried that they may be asked about a previous pregnancy (or abortion) about which their partner has no knowledge. If this is the case, it is best to be candid with the doctor, waiting for a time when he can be spoken to alone. It might be worth asking for a subsequent clinic visit when the specialist can be spoken to privately, when no one else is around. Specialists will not reveal personal or intimate information to anybody else, including one's present partner.

A gynaecological history will be needed, and it helps if the woman comes with the dates of recent menstrual periods. The specialist will also need to know about the frequency of sexual intercourse. A very few people still find these things embarrassing, but obviously how often a couple is having sex is relevant. There is no need to be at all shy about these sorts of details. Every consultant gynaecologist is used to a very wide variety of problems and difficulties, and he or she certainly will not embarrass patients with detailed questions.

Some women are naturally worried about a pelvic examination. Those who find this especially embarrassing should certainly say so. In practice, provided a woman is having regular normal intercourse and there are no uterine abnormalities or an ovarian cyst, remarkably little useful information is gained by an internal examination. This can also be deferred until a subsequent visit, when confidence has been gained. Examination of the man also often gives limited information, unless he has an abnormal sperm count. Even then, most men will be found to be completely normal on examination.

What test are there for infertility?

Infertility tests can really be divided into three types: essential, optional, and the more or less useless. The first group, the 'essential' tests, consists of those which can be done immediately after the first attendance at an infertility clinic or those which take time to organise but are generally essential in nearly all cases of infertility. The second group of 'optional' tests is specialised and is not required in every case, but may be helpful if either (1) pregnancy does not happen fairly soon (normally within six months) after treatment is started, or (2) if the cause of infertility cannot be clearly established. There is also a third group of tests which I term 'uesless'. They may be done, but there is, in my opinion, very little rational basis for them.

No two specialists will do tests in precisely the same order. For example, many will prefer to do a laparoscopy before ordering an X-ray. Others will substitute one kind of test for another. What I have done in this section is to try to lay out my own preferences, with the order of tests that generally makes most sense in my own practice. Tests should be done in a logical fashion and without undue waiting so that they are completed within a reasonable length of time. They should also be explained carefully and the results clearly given.

Essential tests for the man

SPERM COUNT

Male problems are as likely as female ones, and sperm counts, or *semen analyses*, are essential. Three very important points should be remembered. First, a single normal sperm count does not completely exclude a male problem. As we shall see, a man may produce many sperm, freely moving around, but there are subtle problems with them which may prevent fertilisation. Second, an abnormal or low count does not mean that there is necessarily something wrong. Most men produce poor-quality semen from time to time, especially if they are under stress. Good clinics always do several sperm counts before pronouncing on the male's fertility. Third, although a man may have previously fathered a pregnancy he may now be infertile. Men – like women – become infertile after various problems.

HOW IS THE SPERM COUNT DONE?

A good infertility clinic will give clear written instructions about the method of sperm collection they prefer and how soon the semen is needed after collection for analysis. Some clinics prefer a couple not to have had intercourse for three days before a test, though opinions vary about how important this is. Clinics normally provide a little pot together with a form asking for a few basic details. Semen needs to be delivered to the clinic within about two hours of its production. Most men prefer to produce it by masturbation; some like their partners to help them; and others find it easier to produce semen by interrupting intercourse, and ejaculating into the little pot.[18] Don't be embarrassed if you miss the pot, or if not all the semen gets in – just

_____

[18] When I say a little pot, I do mean it. Regrettably, the miserable pot supplied by many clinics is often a little too little, requiring a good eye and a steady hand at a rather inconvenient moment. One husband asked me recently, with an

record this information on the form. Missing part of the semen may make the count abnormally low, but it always can be repeated at a later date. Do not use a condom for sperm collection as most contain substances which kill the sperm.

I recall the redoubtable Miss Ann Croaker, the late Professor McClure Browne's secretary, dealing with one of his new patients from Greece, who spoke no English but reasonable French. Miss Croaker explained in English slowly and clearly that the patient would come for his appointment next Wednesday and that, most important, he must produce the sperm specimen before seeing the Professor. When speaking even louder, invariably her first tactic, did not work, Miss Croaker tried her high-school French. 'Il faut que vous produisez les spermes devant le Professeur.' The Greek gentleman turned pale. 'Mais, Madame, devant le Professeur?' 'Oui, oui, devant le Professeur,' insisted Miss Croaker, whereupon the Greek looked very sheepish indeed and crept from the office. Miss Croaker later realised that 'avant' is rather better than 'devant' if one wants to say 'before' in this context.

WHAT IS A 'NORMAL' SPERM COUNT?

The sperm will be sent to a laboratory where it will be examined under a microscope for the following qualities:

● *Semen volume.* Normally 2–5 millilitres (up to a teaspoonful). If low, he may not be producing enough secretions. Alternatively, part of the sample may not have been collected at ejaculation. A man may think that he is virile if he produces a large volume, but much over 5 millilitres may dilute the sperm too much.

● *Sperm numbers.* Should be greater than 40 million in each millilitre. If below 20 million, there may be a problem. A few men, however, are fully fertile when they produce only 2 or 3 million sperm per millilitre of semen.

● *Sperm motility.* At least 40 per cent of the sperm should be moving. Motility much below this is usually abnormal.

---

apologetic note in his voice, that he wasn't boasting, but was there any chance of something a bit bigger?

● *Normal sperm*. At least 65 per cent of the sperm should look normal under a microscope. If there are many abnormal sperm, there may be a serious problem with their manufacture in the testicles.

● *'Clumping' bacteria, white blood cells*. A good lab will also record whether there is any 'clumping' (i.e. sperm stuck together). This may indicate an infection, or possibly antibodies to the sperm. If this is the case, specialised sperm tests are needed (*see*. p. 143). Many white cells, 'debris', or obvious bacteria may mean infection, making the sperm abnormal.

● *Chemical tests*. Some labs routinely test for certain chemicals such as fructose (*see* p. 144).

● *Antibodies*. Many laboratories routinely test for antibodies that may be attacking the sperm (*see* p. 143).

GETTING SPERM COUNT RESULTS

I strongly recommend that partners should try to go together to get the result of the sperm count. The test result is emotionally very important to both the man and the woman for different reasons, and it can be a considerable burden for the woman to go on her own and find out that her man has a problem. Do not expect a good clinic to give these results over the telephone. For one thing, they can never be sure to whom they are speaking. For another, they cannot give people proper emotional support (if it is needed) over the telephone.

When getting the sperm count results, it is essential to bear in mind that perfectly fertile men may have an abnormal semen test from time to time. A single bad test is simply not diagnostic on its own, so neither partner should be depressed or worried if the first count is below average, or even if there is no sperm present in the sample. This is surprisingly common.

THE POST-COITAL TEST

This is done after sexual intercourse (*coitus*), preferably some 6–36 hours later. The specialist simply takes a sample of fluid from the woman's cervix during a simple internal examination; this is similar to a cervical smear test. He or she then immediately examines the cervical fluid or mucus under a microscope and checks whether sperm are present, and whether the sperm are moving around. This test needs to be performed during the first half of the woman's menstrual cycle, just before ovulation when the mucus is most easily penetrated by the sperm.

Strictly speaking, the post-coital test is not only a test of the man's fertility, but also helps to show that ovulation may be occurring in the woman, that her cervix is healthy and that there is no obvious compatibility problem.

It is a pity that this test is sometimes wrongly neglected as, in the right cases, it gives very useful information, both about the quality of the sperm and about the cervical mucus.

THE REASONS FOR A NEGATIVE POST–COITAL TEST

1. The test has been done too late in the cycle, when ovulation has already occurred, after which cervical mucus production virtually dries up.
2. The test has been done too early in the woman's cycle, before oestrogen is produced in large enough amounts to influence mucus manufacture.
3. The test was done in a cycle when the woman happened not to ovulate.
4. The man just produced poor semen this time.
5. Sperm are not being produced in sufficient quantity, or their quality is not really ideal.
6. The woman has a persistent problem with failure to ovulate.
7. The woman's cervix is abnormal and is therefore producing abnormal, impenetrable mucus.
8. The woman has a scarred or infected cervix which is not producing enough mucus.
9. One partner is producing antibodies which are attacking the sperm.
10. The man is not ejaculating into the vagina properly.

Note that the first four reasons all occur in normal couples and are the most common reasons for a negative test.

MYTHS SURROUNDING THE POST-COITAL TEST

● *A negative test is caused by a tilted (retroverted) uterus.* Wrong: 25 per cent of women have a uterus which is lying in a retroverted position. There is no real evidence that this influences the post-coital test or female fertility.

● *A negative test is caused by the sperm flowing out of the vagina after intercourse.* Wrong. All women, provided there is a reasonable quantity of ejaculate, tend to lose fluid from the vagina after intercourse.

● *The test is negative because sex is happening in the wrong position.* There is no evidence at all that position during intercourse has the slightest influence on fertility.

● *The post-coital test will be negative if it is not done within two or three hours of sexual intercourse.* Wrong. Despite the fact that even many doctors seem to believe this, a properly done test will be positive at least eight hours after intercourse and usually much longer. It may be possible to identify active sperm seventy-two hours after sex. Too many clinics demand that the unfortunate woman must rush up to the hospital immediately after making love so that the test can be performed. This can throw a total unnecessary strain on both partners and many men become totally impotent when such unreasonable demands are made. In such circumstances, it is perfectly justified to refuse a request to rush to the hospital clinic immediately after sex; nor will this refusal invalidate the test.

● *A negative test means that the woman is killing off her partner's sperm.* Wrong. All couples frequently have negative post-coital tests; the test needs to be persistently negative before it can be said that there is any real likelihood that something is wrong.

Essential tests for the woman

TESTING FOR OVULATION

These tests should be organised at the first visit. Good clinics employ more than one test for ovulation to confirm that the ovaries really are working.[19]

BLOOD TEST FOR PROGESTERONE

This is an important and most widely used test for ovulation. Actually, it only gives circumstantial evidence that ovulation has taken place, as it simply measures the amount of the hormone progesterone produced by the ovary – it does not detect whether an egg really left the ovary. As we have seen (*see* Chapter 1) progesterone is one of the female hormones produced by the ovary, mostly during the second half of the cycle.

There are two different ways of expressing these hormone measurements, either 'nmol per litre' (common in Britain) or 'ng per litre' (common in the US). The normal level following ovulation is 30 nmol per litre or 10 ng per litre depending on which measurement is used.

These levels are not reached immediately after ovulation, but about a week later and are maintained for three to five days. This is why it is usual to measure this hormone on the twenty-first day of the menstrual cycle, and why clinics often repeat the blood test two or three days later to confirm that the rise is maintained. The level falls sharply immediately before a period, so a test taken within a day or two of bleeding may be meaningless. This is very important to understand, because many couples become discouraged when they have a low

[19] How often have I written this, and how often have I seen women diagnosed as not ovulating on the basis of one blood test taken on the twenty-first day of the cycle! This kind of lazy diagnosis can hold up effective treatment for months, or even longer.

reading: this result may simply be because the first day of the period occurred earlier or later than expected.

One warning: in people taking the fertility drug clomiphene (Clomid), any measurement of the blood progesterone level can be misleading. Because clomiphene increases the number and size of the follicles in the ovary as well as helping ovulation, a high level of progesterone can be produced even when ovulation has not happened. Unfortunately, many clinics (and, dare I say, doctors) forget this and patients can be lulled into a sense of false security. Therefore, ultrasound tests are much more reliable for those taking Clomid tablets (see p. 149).

TEMPERATURE CHARTS

Temperature charting could actually be put into my third category of tests: those of little value. A great many books, and some clinics, seem to place great importance on temperature charting. However, because it just might be helpful for a month or two when starting tests, here's how to do it.

A standard fertility temperature chart should be collected from the clinic, or bought from a chemist. Each morning, the temperature should be taken with a clinical thermometer (bought also from a chemist's shop) throughout the cycle. This should be done first thing on waking, before getting out of bed, drinking the cup of tea invariably brought by an attentive partner, or smoking a cigarette. The temperature should be taken by placing the thermometer under the tongue for at least one minute.[20] As soon as the temperature has been measured the result should be recorded on the temperature chart which of course is always immediately to hand on the bedside table.

---

[20] The French, for reasons I have never understood, advise taking the temperature by inserting the thermometer into the rectum. There seems to be a popular belief, apparently held by some continental physicians, that things inserted rectally are always more effective.

The pitfalls of temperature charts

While it is true that a woman's body temperature rises slightly after ovulation (probably because the increased levels of progesterone increase her metabolism), many perfectly normally ovulating women never have an appreciable change. People who are charting their temperature are often wrongly disappointed and distressed. On the other hand, some women who are not ovulating effectively do notice some rise in temperature after the mid-cycle, and may be misled into thinking their ovaries are working properly.

Finally, but most important, some women are led to believe that their temperature chart will tell them when they are at their most fertile and use the chart to time intercourse. As we have already seen, the best time to conceive is by making love 12–48 hours before ovulation – this is, of course, before the temperature starts rising. It is true that, just before ovulation, some women experience an apparent fall in temperature; some 'authorities' recommend using this to time sex. Unfortunately, there are a great many reasons why the temperature may fall and this is a most unreliable sign.

The objections to keeping temperature charts

● They are generally very unreliable and can be misleading, particularly in women with irregular cycles.
● They are a constant reminder that one is desperately trying to get pregnant.
● They can be infuriatingly inconvenient, especially for those who are travelling or on holiday, or busy working, particularly on night shifts.
● They encourage many couples to make love to order, destroying spontaneity. This, for my money, is the most important objection. You are convinced, from the drop in temperature this morning, that tonight's the night. Your husband comes home from a row with his boss, dog-tired. You forget to put the cat out, or burn the soup. He doesn't feel sexy.

You end up half trying to have intercourse, but certainly not making love. Both of you finish by feeling bad. This, a not untypical scenario, repeated in different ways each month, can be extremely demoralising.

The advantages of temperature charting

● They are a very cheap way of testing that ovulation may be occurring, and avoid hospital tests.
● They give a chance to do something which might help.
● They help people take some control of the problem away from doctors.
● They are quite a good way of keeping a record of period dates.
● For a few women, they are not inconvenient and are quite reliable.

Those who do decide to do a temperature chart should set a time limit on the number of months for this experiment. It is worth also getting supporting evidence of the chart's reliability by alternative, simultaneous tests. Finally, it really is not terribly healthy to time one's sex life by using a temperature chart.

ENDOMETRIAL BIOPSY

An endometrial biopsy is a tiny piece of the uterine lining (endometrium), examined under the microscope. Provided the biopsy is done during the second half of the menstrual cycle, it helps decide whether or not the uterine lining has been exposed and responded to the progesterone that is normally produced by the ovary after ovulation.

How an endometrial biopsy is done

The best time is from the eighteenth day of a twenty-eight-day cycle up to the time of menstruation. The cervix is cleaned after simple examination. A small pipe is inserted through it and a tiny scraping of the lining of the uterus is removed within seconds. This can cause brief discomfort – a little cramp-like period pain. Because a few women feel unhappy or frightened about the discomfort occasionally experienced it is common for clinics (my own included) to delay this test until the patient comes for laparoscopy under anaesthesia.

TESTING THE TUBES AND UTERUS

THE HYSTEROSALPINGOGRAM

The hysterosalpingogram (or HSG, for short) is an X-ray of the uterus and Fallopian tubes. Sadly, it is a rather neglected test and some doctors even believe that the need for it has been replaced by laparoscopy. In fact, a properly done HSG gives information impossible to get by other methods. During the test, a little dye is placed into the uterus and X-rays are taken. The tubes can be viewed to see whether they are open or not, but more importantly, the quality of the shadow on the X-ray can give very good detail of the outline of the inside of the uterus – very difficult to achieve by other methods and the shadows produced by the tubes themselves give a good idea of not only tubal blockage but whether there is extensive scarring unsuitable for surgical treatment.

It is quite important that the specialist looks at the actual X-rays rather than the report which comes from the radiologist. One patient of mine, who lived abroad, came to see me with the following report:

> Mrs S S: X-ray of baby bag reveals creating of spray alright with no rocks. Egg basket poor visualized with good hatsatsora shadowed by agenj lulaot liquid observed in both trumpets but not captivated and query spilling but it's not clear from which side.

I like 'not clear from which side'. Fortunately, the X-rays themselves were a bit more informative.

When should a hysterosalpingogram be done?

We organise an HSG as soon as we can after the first clinic visit. Then, when the couple return for the first follow-up, we already have valuable information about the quality of the tubes and the uterus. There are certain situations, though, when the HSG may be better done after a laparoscopy (*see* p. 139) – for example, when one knows one has some form of tubal damage.

It is unwise to have any X-ray of the abdomen if there is even the slightest possibility of being pregnant. Because of this, it is best for the HSG to be performed during the first half of the cycle, before ovulation. If it is difficult to get an appointment for an HSG in the first two weeks of the cycle, it is perfectly reasonable to have the X-ray more than two weeks after a period, provided some effective contraception is used (a condom, for example) during that month. The HSG should not be done during the period itself, because it is thought that this may be a cause of endometriosis.

Having an X-ray

The doctor will normally first do a simple internal examination on the X-ray couch. He then inserts a small tube through the cervix. This tube is thin – the part which actually fits inside the cervix is no large than a ball-point pen refill. This may cause fleeting discomfort but certainly no worse than that experienced with a period. A small amount of dye is gently injected into the uterus, and the progress of the dye can be seen on a television screen and X-rays can be taken. Usually about six of these are taken, and the procedure takes ten minutes. This procedure does not require hospital admission or an anaesthetic and is painless in most cases.

While it is true that the HSG has a bad reputation for causing discomfort, this is now quite unjustified. If modern techniques are used (especially the newer, less irritant X-ray dyes), the doctor is gentle and the dye injected slowly, most women do not realise the test has started or finished. However, because many are nervous about the test and a very few do have

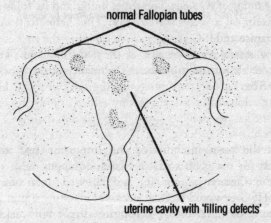

Hysterosalpingogram (HSG). Special X-ray dye has been injected through the cervix (at the bottom of the picture), and the inside of the uterine cavity and Fallopian tubes are outlined by the dye. In this woman the tubes are normal and open, but there are areas in the uterine cavity that have not filled – possibly due to fibroids.

crampy discomfort, it is sensible to be accompanied at the X-ray appointment by a partner or friend. They can give moral support and a bit of company on the way home if there is any soreness. Persistent pain after the HSG (particularly hours later) is definitely abnormal and if this is experienced, the hospital should be contacted for advice, no matter how late at night.

What information does a hysterosalpingogram give?

Laparoscopy is just as good, if not better, at telling whether the tubes are open. Nevertheless, HSG gives unique information about:

● *The inside of the uterus*. It is very good as showing adhesions inside the womb, as well as fibroids, adenomyosis and polyps.

● *The area where the tubes join the uterus*. This area, the internal plumbing of which is exceptionally delicate and small, is poorly seen at laparoscopy. The HSG gives an idea whether there is any scar tissue in this area, or polyps in the tube itself.

● *The lining of the tube.* The tubal lining and its folds show up very nicely on a well-taken X-ray. This helps to decide if the tubes are scarred.

● *How scarred the tubes are*, if they are blocked. This gives important information about whether surgery is worth considering.

LAPAROSCOPY

This is the most informative and important test for female infertility. If I was on a desert island (equipped with a modern operating theatre, of course) and allowed only one test for infertility, this would be it. It involves inserting a thin telescope into the abdominal cavity through a small hole made in the navel. To get a good view, a little carbon dioxide gas is first passed into the abdomen. This separates all the organs and makes them easier to see. The telescope is no thicker than a fountain pen, but due to the remarkable development of modern optics, the view is superb. Photographs of very high quality can be taken via the telescope – a facility which more and more surgeons are using. The surgeon can inspect the uterus through the laparoscope, test the tubes to see if they are open or scarred on the outside, and look at the ovaries. It is true to say that laparoscopy – far more than test-tube baby treatment or any other development – has been the single most revolutionary advance in infertility diagnosis and treatment.

What does a laparoscopy involve?

In general, it is best done in the second half of the cycle, so that the surgeon can examine the ovaries to see if ovulation happened.

Although a few surgeons do laparoscopy under local anaesthesia, a general anaesthetic with the patient asleep is usual. Laparoscopy requires an overnight stay in hospital. A few centres now do laparoscopy as a day-care procedure, usually to cut costs.

Laparoscopy takes 20–40 minutes and carries no serious

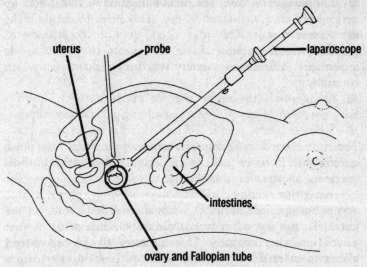

Laparoscopy. Carbon dioxide gas has already been injected into the tummy to separate the organs so that the surgeon gets a good view down the telescope.

risk. On waking there will normally be two small dressings on the abdomen. One covers a single stitch in the navel, the other a tiny hole near the pubic hairline. This second hole is used to place any fine probes into the abdominal cavity which may be required to get a better view. Most people have very little discomfort and no pain after laparoscopy; others may feel a bit sore. A very few woman feel distinctly unwell and need to rest in bed for twenty-four hours. The commonest side-effects are:

● Soreness in the abdomen (usually not at all bad).

● Soreness or pain in one or other shoulder. This may seem a strange place to feel discomfort when all the surgery is in the lower abdomen. It is due to carbon dioxide gas irritating the nerves to the abdominal lining. These are the same nerves that supply the shoulder area, hence the discomfort.

● Vaginal bleeding. This may occur because the surgeon has manipulated the cervix during the injection of the dye to check the tubes. The bleeding is usually heavy enough to warrant wearing a sanitary towel for two or three days, and it may go on longer.

● A sore throat. This may occur because the anaesthetist placed a breathing tube down the throat to ensure a safe anaesthetic. This soreness rarely lasts longer than twenty-four hours.

● Sleeplessness the night after or vivid dreams. This is a frequent effect of any procedure involving general anaesthesia.

● Sickness. Some people feel sick after having an anaesthetic. Fewer do these days because the action of the drugs is so much gentler than in times past. Special drugs can be given to those prone to sickness after anaesthesia.

After laparoscopy done on a day-care basis, people usually rest in hospital for four to six hours and then go home; because dizziness after any procedure is common, the homeward journey is best in the company of a friend or relative. Avoid wetting the areas covered by the dressings for forty-eight hours. Most surgeons put an absorbable stitch in the navel and this will usually dissolve after two to four weeks.

What can be gained from laparoscopy?

● It is the best way of determining whether the tubes are damaged.

● It is extremely valuable in seeing if there are any adhesions in the abdominal cavity (see p. 185).

● It gives a direct view of the ovaries and, provided the laparoscopy is done in the second half of the cycle, the surgeon can see whether there has been recent ovulation.

● It is the best way to detect endometriosis.

● It gives an excellent view of the outside of the uterus and may help to detect fibroids or a congenital problem in the womb.

● It is a useful aid to see if there are other diseases affecting the ovaries, such as cysts, or other diseases in the abdominal cavity.

● After laparoscopy, rather more women immediately conceive than would be expected by chance. About 15 per cent of our patients with open tubes conceive within three months of laparoscopy. The reason for this is not clear but may be due to the action of flushing the tubes with dye.

Optional tests for the man

The following tests may be helpful if more than one sperm count is abnormal or low.

SEPARATION TEST (SWIM TEST)

This tests sperm function. Available in specialist centres, it involves placing the semen in special fluids to see how many sperm can swim properly. The normal sperm separate from the abnormal ones, giving an idea of how many may be capable of fertilising an egg.

One problem with this test is that the semen needs to be quite fresh. Most clinics like the semen to be produced in the hospital, but few hospitals offer adequate facilities for producing semen, and most men have to produce semen in the nearest lavatory. In some hospitals, a proper bedroom is available; very often this is oversubscribed, resulting in the embarrassment of the men queuing up to use the 'facilities'. If ever a man needs a sense of humour and perspective during infertility tests, now is the time.

COMPUTER SPERM MOTILITY TESTS

An increasing number of laboratories are using computerised measurement of sperm function and motility. Sperm are observed under a microscope to which a television camera is attached; their movements are digitised by a computer – usually an IBM with extra memory chips – and then the quality of the movement of individual sperm is assessed. This may be helpful in assessing how 'good' the sperm are. This test is more widely available in the United States than in Britain, partly because of technological enthusiasm. Computer imaging equipment for sperm counting and measurement is beyond the pocket of most NHS units. However, there is no good evidence that digitised computer sperm counting is much improvement over simpler methods, although they are likely to be increasingly used in future.

ANTIBODY TESTING

Some men certainly produce antibodies which identify the sperm (or parts of them, such as the heads or the tails) as foreign protein. This results in the sperm sticking together, or being deficient in other ways, particularly in being less able to propel themselves around. Two tests may be done to detect antibodies: the MAR test, done on the semen; the Kibrick test, done on blood. Unless the levels of antibody are clearly high, there is doubt about the relevance of these tests. Sperm clumping can also be caused by infection.

SPERM CULTURE

If an infection is suspected, some laboratories culture the semen to try to identify the bacterium responsible before antibiotic treatment is undertaken. These cultures tend to be quite unreliable, which is why they are by no means done routinely.

FRUCTOSE MEASUREMENT

If there are no sperm in the semen, there may be a blockage either above or below the seminal vesicles. The seminal vesicles produce fructose, a simple sugar which is easily measured in semen. If the semen is low in fructose, this suggests that the blockage is below the seminal vesicles, which helps direct a surgeon where to look.

SPLIT EJACULATE TEST

During ejaculation, the first part of the semen tends to be richer in sperm, even when the sperm count is a bit low. This 'concentrated' semen may be worth collecting for subsequent artificial insemination (*see* Chapter 9). The split ejaculate test helps evaluate this. It is devilishly hard to do, as it involves the man juggling between two collecting pots – usually while masturbating. Even performers at the Moscow State Circus would find this difficult. Sometimes a partner can be very helpful here. Infertility treatment is sometimes a remarkable way of overcoming life's little sensitivities.

HAMSTER TEST

This involves testing sperm to see if they penetrate the eggs of a golden hamster. A simple sperm count does not give a good idea about whether sperm function normally. One theoretical way of getting around this is to see how they react in contact with eggs from other mammals but only the hamster egg is a reasonably good model. Prepared semen is mixed with hamster eggs and the number of eggs penetrated by sperm is counted. (Rest assured that a hamster egg penetrated by human sperm is completely incapable of developing into an embryo). If no eggs are penetrated, this suggests that the sperm function is inadequate. Recent evidence suggests that this test is not very reliable and so it has been largely abandoned.[21]

HUMAN ZONA PENETRATION TEST

The ability of a sperm to penetrate the zona (the 'shell') of the egg is an important function. To test this, the sperm can be

---

[21] This is gratifying because previously the method of collecting fresh eggs from hamsters required the sacrifice of these engaging creatures.

mixed with dead human eggs obtained from a 'spare' ovary removed during hysterectomy. If sperm penetrate the outer layer, there is no risk of an embryo being formed as the egg is dead. It is presently available in only a few research centres.

HUMAN ZONA ATTACHMENT TEST

Another rather similar test involves counting the number of sperm which attach to the zona (one of the first stages of fertilising, before actual penetration of the zona itself occurs). This is also experimental but promising, and has given some useful information about sperm function of a rather non-specific nature.

HORMONE TESTS

A very few men with low sperm counts have a hormonal problem. Occasionally, the pituitary gland may not be producing enough LH or FSH (the same hormones that regulate a woman's menstrual cycle), and this is measurable and treatable. Conversely, high levels of these hormones suggest that no treatment is likely to be of assistance. Measurement of the male hormone *testosterone* may also help decide whether the testicles are capable of working normally. Sometimes the hormone *prolactin* produced by the pituitary gland in both men and women is also measured. In women it stimulates the production of breast milk but in men this function is irrelevant. Although in rare cases prolactin may be abnormally high its level in men is of dubious importance.

TESTICULAR BIOPSY

This is done by a surgeon who removes a tiny sliver of tissue from a testicle. This requires an anaesthetic and an overnight hospital stay. Microscopic examination of the tissue sample will reveal whether the testis is producing sperm or not. If it is not producing sperm properly, the fact that there is no real treatment may have to be faced. Testicular biopsy is really only worth doing in a few cases.

TESTICULAR X-RAYS (VASOGRAPHY)

This may be done at the time of a testicular biopsy. A little dye is squirted into the vas deferens, and the epididymis may also be examined at the same time. This may establish whether or not there is a blockage which may be worth operating upon. These X-rays are very pretty – men who have this done should be sure to ask to have a look.

THERMOGRAPHY

This is used in some centres, mostly in the United States, to assess the temperature of the testicles. The man places his testicles over a heat-sensitive plate, which then changes colour (like the paper thermometers bought in chemists' shops). If the plate turns blue, this means that one of the testicles is hot and that there may be a varicocoele present (see p. 117). I am not convinced that this test is particularly useful. Thermography is at least totally painless, and the pretty colours are fun.

KARYOTYPE (CHROMOSOME) TEST

For this, the blood is usually tested. Some men who produce very few or no sperm have a genetic (chromosomal) problem. A chromosome count can reveal this. Unfortunately, there is no treatment if this is the problem.

IN VITRO FERTILISATION (IVF)

'Washed' sperm can be mixed with a live egg taken from an ovary just before ovulation. This is, in fact, the test-tube baby process. If an embryo develops, this is, of course, the best proof that the sperm are capable of normal activity. Any embryo that is obtained can be put back into the woman's uterus, where it may develop into a baby. In many ways, this is the ultimate test of sperm function; the reason it is not done more often is because it is very expensive. It is, of course, available at IVF centres.

An optional test for both partners

CROSSED MUCUS PENETRATION TEST (MUCUS HOSTILITY TEST)

This may be used when the man's sperm count is more or less normal, but the post-coital test is repeatedly negative. It involves examining under a microscope either a sample of the man's sperm combined with cervical mucus from a donor, or donor sperm mixed with the woman's mucus. This may help decide whether it is the male or female partner who is producing antibodies that are killing off the sperm.

Optional tests for the woman

These tests are done by an increasing number of clinics, particularly if the cause of infertility is unclear, or if a subtle problem with ovulation is suspected.

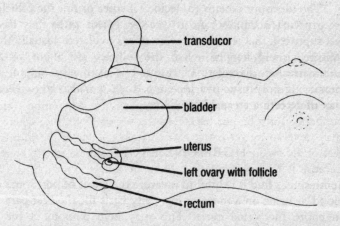

Ultrasound examination. The sound waves are sent from the transducer to structures in the abdominal cavity, where they bounce back to the transducer again. These reflections are then translated into a picture on a TV screen.

OVARIAN ULTRASOUND

This is very useful – so useful that many specialists try it first. Ultrasonic sound waves are aimed at the ovaries through the abdominal wall or the vagina, and the echoes obtained can be picked up and displayed on a television screen. It is very similar to the sonar used on ships. Modern ultrasound allows very precise measurement (to the nearest millimetre) of many structures inside the abdomen. Ultrasound works best through water, which is an excellent conductor of sound. This is why abdominal ultrasound is performed when the bladder is really full – it gives a better picture of the ovaries, which lie just behind the bladder. Some well-equipped clinics also have vaginal ultrasound where a small ultrasound probe can be put in the vagina and an excellent view of the ovaries obtained. This has many advantages; filling the bladder full enough for abdominal ultrasound can be very uncomfortable.[22]

[22] Ultrasound is one of the great advances in recent medicine. Much credit for

The ultrasound helps to decide whether or not the follicles are growing normally, and it can also detect when they have just ruptured: that is, when a woman has ovulated. Usually this rupture should happen when the follicles are about 18–20 millimetres in diameter. Ultrasound is also very helpful in identifying polycystic ovaries (*see* p. 105). It is also an excellent way of detecting an early pregnancy.

HORMONE PROFILES

Some clinics find it helpful to measure the levels of hormones in blood or urine on a more or less daily basis for the best part of an entire menstrual cycle. This may help pinpoint a subtle hormone abnormality, which may be responsible for failure to ovulate properly. It is customary to measure the hormones oestrogen, LH and progesterone, and compare the results with the levels of a group of women known to be ovulating normally.

MEASUREMENT OF LH AND FSH

This is often useful if there is an ovulatory problem. If the levels of these two hormones are low, pituitary hormone treatment may be indicated. If the levels are a little raised, the ovaries may be polycystic. Rarely, LH and FSH may be very high indeed; unfortunately, this suggests that the ovaries may not have any eggs in them and a menopausal state is likely.

TESTOSTERONE MEASUREMENT

Raised levels of male hormone (which women also produce normally) suggest that one may not be ovulating. This may be

---

its development is due to Professor Ian Donald, who worked at Hammersmith before moving to Glasgow. Against the usual opposition and sarcasm, he persisted with his ultrasound transducer and Cathode ray tube, until the introduction of computing made his instrument into the device which revolutionised obstetrics, gynaecology, and much general medicine. He should have won a Nobel Prize.

seen with certain types of polycystic ovary syndrome. It can also, very rarely, be associated with other diseases of the ovaries or the adrenal glands.

PROLACTIN MEASUREMENT

This hormone is frequently raised, but infrequently causes a problem. Unfortunately, many women become very alarmed when told they have a high prolactin level. It is worth remembering that if the *progesterone* level is normal and consistent with ovulation, a raised prolactin level is irrelevant. A high prolactin level only needs treating (with drugs, usually) if there is definite evidence that ovulation is not occurring.

SKULL X-RAY AND EYE TEST

If prolactin levels are raised, this may be because there is an enlarged pituitary gland which is overactive but not producing LH or FSH. Very rarely, this swelling can be a benign tumour. An X-ray of the skull in the region of the pituitary gland may detect such a problem. Because the visual fields (how far around one can see) can be affected, the doctor may want to do an eye test as well.

THYROID HORMONE MEASUREMENT

Very frequently measured, this is very infrequently the cause of failure to ovulate. Thyroid problems cause less than 1 per cent of infertility due to ovulation failure in most clinics.

KARYOTYPE (CHROMOSOME) TEST

Just as men with a chromosomal abnormality may not produce normal sperm, so might women not produce normal eggs if they have a similar problem. The blood can be tested, and the result usually takes at least three to four weeks. These abnormalities are rare.

EXTRA TESTS FOR THE TUBES OR UTERUS

These may be helpful, but many centres do not have facilities for them.

HYSTEROSCOPY

A small telescope – called an *hysteroscope* – is passed into the uterus. It is usually done under quick general anaesthetic on a day visit to the hospital. Hysteroscopy is excellent at detecting abnormalities suspected after an HSG, such as polyps, uterine fibroids, a congenital abnormality or any adhesions which may scar the lining of the uterus. The hysteroscope can also be used to treat some of these conditions by guiding the fine scissors or other instruments inside the uterus.

TUBOSCOPY

A few specialists may wish to examine the inside of the Fallopian tubes, using a fine telescope. This is usually inserted through the abdomen wall while under general anaesthetic. A telescope, usually about 3 millimetres in diameter, is used to inspect the inside of the ovarian end of the tube. It is helpful because it aids in diagnosing areas of scarring or fine adhesions inside the tubes.

FALLOPOSCOPY

This is somewhat similar to tuboscopy, but can be done as an out-patient procedure because the telescope is passed into the tube from below, through the vagina and uterus. It is a very thin, fragile telescope about the thickness of a piece of linen thread, and gives a view of the uterine end of the tube. This telescope is usually attached to a TV camera and the result viewed on a screen. Because the diameter of the telescope is so slender, the resolution (quality of picture) is not as good as that seen using tuboscopy.

TESTS OF DUBIOUS VALUE

TUBAL INSUFFLATION

My own pet aversion is tubal insufflation. Regrettably, some patients are still offered this, mostly by very old-fashioned doctors, and I would suggest that women firmly refuse. This test involves injecting carbon dioxide gas under pressure through a metal pipe attached to the cervix into the uterus.[23] If the pressure does not rise above a certain level or the doctor can hear the gas bubbling through with a stethoscope or the unfortunate woman experiences pain in the tip of her shoulder, this is taken as evidence that gas is getting through the uterus and tubes. This test is a museum piece. When it was invented – in 1919 by Dr Rubin of New York – it was reasonable because there was nothing better. It is painful, somewhat dangerous and very unreliable. The apparatus used to perform it is very beautiful to look at and would be best housed in a locked glass case in a mahogany cabinet.

[23] The late Dr Green-Armytage (G-A as he was called), a formidable and terrifying man, ran one of the first infertility clinics in Britain, before the Second World War. Once his junior house-surgeon timorously tried to do this test in the out-patient clinic at Hammersmith. Having caused the stoical patient considerable pain for fifteen minutes, he crept out of the clinic to inform G-A that he could not get the pipe attached to the cervix. Cursing at his incompetence, the boss strode in and spent another agonising fifteen minutes before finally succeeding, but the test was negative. G-A called the clinic Sister commanding that while the pipe was in position, the unfortunate patient should go to X-ray to get some dye injected down the pipe. Sister sent for a trolley for the patient, whereupon G-A shouted to her to stop mollycoddling the woman, saying that she could walk the half-mile to the X-ray Department. Sister replied that no patient of hers was walking for ten minutes with that 'ruddy great thing between her legs', to which G-A responded, 'Madam, I have walked around for fifty-two years with this ruddy great thing between my legs.' Nevertheless, the patient went on the trolley.

D & C (DILATATION AND CURETTAGE)

Some women are still brought into hospital for a 'womb scrape' if they are having difficulty in conceiving. Though harmless, it is valueless unless done at the time of a laparoscopy, when an endometrial biopsy is taken. It is performed because of a myth which suggests that it is easier to conceive after a D & C. There is no truth in this.

MEASUREMENT OF TRACE ELEMENTS, VITAMINS, HAIR TESTING

There are a few private clinics preying on the desperation of infertile couples by offering tests of unproven or spurious value. A typical clinic will charge £20 or £30 per test to examine a small lock of hair for various metals or other substances. Usually the result comes back showing an absence of zinc, magnesium, or too much potassium, or some equally irrelevant compound – pure hocus-pocus.

CHAPTER NINE

Routine Infertility Treatments

In Chapter 2 we looked at simple ways of helping oneself to get pregnant. We also saw the limitations of 'self-help'. Here we look at the various medical treatments available, what they have to offer, what they involve, and what kind of success rates may be expected. While obviously, as a doctor, I am biased in favour of active medical treatment, I have to say that all infertility treatment is limited. There are a few points worth remembering:

● Medical treatment is all very well, but many couples find it a huge help to feel that they have some control over the process.

● Many infertile couples achieve a pregnancy while undergoing no active treatment. Very few women, and only a few men, are ever completely sterile (even if treatment has failed).

Suzanne and Jeremy came to see me in February 1992. They had experienced sixteen years of infertility. They had already been seen in four different clinics elsewhere and exhaustive, and sometimes repeated tests, had never shown a satisfactory cause for the infertility. Many different treatments including GIFT and IVF (*see* Chapter 11) had been tried. We spent some time talking and arranged to do one or two specialised tests which I thought might just be worth while, though I wasn't fully convinced. We arranged a follow-up appointment for March, four weeks later.

Suzanne did one of the blood tests, Jeremy one of the special sperm tests. They never did the other investigations I ordered, because her next period did not come. At the March visit I was able to show Suzanne the results of her positive pregnancy test. They were absurdly and delightfully grateful to me, though of course, I had done nothing.

Suzanne and Jeremy's experience is not that uncommon. It is a good reminder that infertility is seldom absolute, and that we doctors have only limited powers.

● All active treatments for infertility are limited in success. Statistics from infertility clinics (including centres doing test-tube baby treatment) clearly show that *only 35 per cent of patients conceive as a result of the treatment they undergo.*

● It is, therefore, impossible for any doctor to predict the result of treatment. There are two things that few candid or truthful doctors can ever say to you:

1. 'There is no chance of you conceiving.'
2. 'This treatment will almost certainly help you have a baby.'

Treatment for the man

Male infertility is very difficult to treat. All methods for improving sperm counts are extremely unreliable. Worse still, if the sperm quality is poor, treatment to improve it may be totally useless. The basic problem is that we still do not understand why some sperm are healthy and others not.

One of the greatest difficulties is that there is a peculiar paradox. If sperm are being produced at all, however few, there is always the possibility of success. Only one sperm is needed to produce a baby. This means that sometimes men with an apparently hopelessly low sperm count may eventually get their partners pregnant.

To add to the difficulties of prediction, some men produce very poor sperm for some years and then, quite suddenly and often without reason, start to produce much better quality sperm. Very frequently, if they are under treatment at the time, the improvement in sperm count is gratefully attributed to the therapy being given, but this may not be the true reason.

Even though simple remedies are unlikely to influence the

complex events that contribute to sperm function, there is some real hope. Various measures are undoubtedly of value in improving male fertility, and some of them work quite dramatically.

GENERAL HEALTH MEASURES

There is moderately good evidence that an improvement in general health may make a difference to male infertility. Many fertile men are prone to poor sperm counts, which may make them at least temporarily infertile. If the sperm count is marginal or low, certain health rules may maximise the chances of a baby. For example, the hazards described on pp. 119–20 are relatively simple to correct, and this can be much more effective than other treatments with drugs. Perseverance with these suggestions is undoubtedly quite valuable, but it takes about seventy days to make a sperm so the sperm count may not actually improve much for the first four months or so.

LOSE EXCESS WEIGHT

Losing excessive body weight by a suitable diet can be helpful. It is better to reduce gradually, losing around 2 pounds (1 kg) each week.

STOP SMOKING

Smoking is bad for fertility. Anyone with a poor sperm count who smokes more than eight or ten cigarettes a day may make any other treatment useless. I encourage all IVF patients to give up. Heavy smokers cannot expect their sperm count to return to normal immediately on giving up the habit.

Richard, a thirty-three-year-old salesman, and his wife Jean came to see me after they had failed to have a baby after eleven years. She ovulated rather poorly and had been taking fertility drugs for seven years without a pregnancy. His sperm counts were always low, and artificial insemination had been tried many times without success. We measured his count four times in four successive months. The number of sperm per millilitre varied between 4 million and 9 million, the sperm's motility was never more than 30 per cent and usually about 40 per cent of the sperm showed some microscopic abnormality. I advised Richard to lose 20 pounds (9 kg) and to stop smoking – at that time he was smoking 35–40 cigarettes a day. His work involved driving a great deal, but he didn't feel he could alter this much.

I saw him three months later. He had cut down to four cigarettes a day and had lost over 14 pounds (6 kg). He continued with his normal work but was now exercising twice weekly for the first time in years. His sperm count on the day of his appointment was 56 million per millilitre and 50 per cent of the sperm were moving normally although about 30 per cent still showed some abnormality in shape. His sperm count remained at this level two months later. Five weeks after the second of these counts, his wife had a positive pregnancy test, and at the time of writing, Jean is in her second pregnancy.

KEEP ALCOHOL TO A MINIMUM

With everyone having a different reaction to drink, it is impossible to state precise limits. Men with depressed sperm counts shouldn't drink more than 2–3 pints (1.5 litres) of beer daily. More than half a bottle of wine a day may be harmful. I have it on good authority that if the wine is from Burgundy and bottled by a good shipper, it will have an undoubted tonic effect. Spirits may be more harmful, and two or three measures a day are enough.

DRUGS

Medically prescribed drugs need to be discussed with the doctor. Obviously, drugs that are important to health cannot be stopped, but a change or a different dosage might be helpful.

AVOID EXCESSIVE EXERCISE

Regular marathon running or daily vigorous games of squash may be unwise. When physical training is taken too far, it is sensible to ease off for a while to see if the sperm count improves. One friend of mine, a regular marathon runner, found it very difficult to cut down on the amount of exercise he was doing even though his sperm counts were persistently low. However, within a few weeks of reducing the amount of exercise he did by half, the sperm count returned to virtually normal values – and his wife became pregnant three weeks later.

REDUCING TESTICULAR TEMPERATURE

Men are frequently told to take cold baths and wear loose-fitting underwear. There is very limited logic behind these suggestions. The testicles hang outside the body in the scrotum. It seems that sperm production is best when the testicles are several degrees cooler than 98.4° F (37°C) and it is just possible that close-fitting underwear, such as Y-fronts, causes overheating. Because of this, some doctors recommend men with low sperm counts to wear loose boxer shorts and even bathe the scrotum daily in very cold water.[24] There is really no proof that any of this will help, and some couples feel it adds an element of torture to what is already an unpleasant situation. On the other hand, it does no harm and may be worth a go if only because it means that everything possible is being done. Wearing loose-fitting underwear makes reasonable sense, and it seems a good idea to avoid very hot baths and saunas. Readers may be interested to know that, in some parts of the world (especially Japan), hot baths have been used as a method of male contraception.

---

[24] One patient of mine was informed by a Harley Street doctor to use ice-packs on his testicles. He made a virtue of supposed necessity by getting his partner to slap the ice-packs on to his scrotum at the moment of orgasm. Apparently, this greatly increased his pleasure; it did little for his fertility.

DRUG TREATMENTS

Drug treatment is extremely limited in value. I think that many drugs are given largely because patients expect them and because it is much easier for the doctor to give some treatment rather than to be brutally frank. At least 200 different drugs have been prescribed over the years to improve sperm quality and numbers. This says it all because, if there were a proven drug, there would have been far less 'blunderbuss' treatment. The truth is that, except in a few specific cases, drugs are not likely to make much difference. This is, of course, depressing news, but it is important to recognise the problem from the outset. This will avoid wasting a lot of time by taking different but equally ineffective drugs. It also will allow people to take proper decisions about what they should both do about the infertility.

The following drugs are frequently tried:

TESTOSTERONE (MALE HORMONE)

Large doses of testosterone actually reduce the sperm count, so there is no point in long-term testosterone treatment. Some men, though, have a 'rebound' effect. A short course of treatment with large doses of testosterone (given usually by injection) temporarily suppresses their sperm production. When the drug is stopped, the testicles may 'rebound' and there are claims that as many as 50 per cent of men will have a marked improvement in sperm count, though this effect will last only a short time.

MESTEROLONE (PRO-VIRON)

This is a synthetic by-product of testosterone and is claimed to improve sperm motility and possibly sperm number. It is probably the most widely used drug for male infertility, but there is disappointingly little hard evidence that it improves fertility. We have used this drug extensively for very many years on large numbers of men; although some have shown improvements in sperm count, it is quite possible that this improved by itself. Very few of the men taking mesterolone have got their partners pregnant, probably no more than would have done so by chance.

GONADOTROPHINS (PITUITARY HORMONES FSH AND LH)

These may be given by injection (Pergonal or Humegon). Alternatively, LH may be given alone, usually as HCG (human chorionic gonadotrophin; brand names Pregnyl, Profasi). Claims have been made that, because these compounds increase the activity of the testicles, sperm counts rather than motility may improve. In any case, their effect seems variable. They have been proved effective only for men with a pituitary abnormality, when normal production of FSH is decreased. There is some recent evidence that pure FSH may be helpful in large, prolonged doses. On the whole, however, these drugs are generally not justified unless there is a definite and well-defined hormone problem.

CLOMIPHENE (CLOMID) AND TAMOXIFEN (TAMOFEN)

These are mostly used to stimulate the pituitary in women (*see* below); they also affect the ovary and uterus directly – sometimes unfavourably. They have occasionally been used to raise testosterone production by the testicles in the hope of improving the sperm count. Success has been very variable. We have used clomiphene and tamoxifen a lot in the past but have never been convinced that anyone we have given them to has benefited. We have now almost abandoned using this group of drugs for male infertility.

ANTIBIOTICS

There is little doubt that if there is an infection impairing sperm motility or quality, the chance of fertilisation is reduced. Taking antibiotics may solve this problem as sperm motility often improves when any infection in the male genital tract is effectively treated. Treatment is usually needed for four to six weeks.

IMMUNE THERAPY WITH STEROIDS

If sperm counts are poor because of antibodies to the sperm, drugs may just be helpful. Corticosteroids are most commonly used, either prednisolone or ACTH. These drugs may be taken intermittently for several months and in quite high doses, and can be effective only if the testicles are not irreversibly damaged. They are not without quite serious side-effects, including stomach bleeding, mental depression, weight gain and a general feeling of being unwell. The usual practice is to give high doses of prednisolone for seven days or so each month to coincide with the woman's fertile period; such quick 'in-and-out' treatment doesn't usually give time for any side-effects to develop. Whatever the situation, nobody should take steroids for more than three or four months. It is claimed that about half of all men with antibodies may be helped by these drugs – that is, about 3 or 4 per cent of all infertile men.

The sperm can also be 'washed' in specially prepared solutions. The 'washed' sperm can then be inseminated into the cervix with a little syringe. So far, this has had only limited success.

SURGERY

REMOVING A VARICOCOELE

Surgical correction of a varicose varicocoele, or vein in a testicle, is very simple but there are conflicting opinions about its value. The problem is that about 20 per cent of both fertile and infertile men have a varicocoele and this seems no disadvantage to a fertile man. It is, however, thought that there is more chance of infertility if there is abnormal bloodflow in these varicose veins.

The operation involves tying off the abnormal vessels

(ligation) or blocking them, usually with a chemical injection. If the injection method is used, a local anaesthetic is generally all that is needed. The procedure is neither painful nor dangerous and requires at most no more than one night in hospital. X-rays may be taken during surgery to confirm that the veins are effectively blocked. Some surgeons claim that at least 70 per cent of treated men show an improvement in sperm count within three months. Others are less optimistic and some have not found that ligation of a varicocoele produces any improvement.

UNBLOCKING THE TUBING

The tubes that carry sperm are very tiny. For example, the epididymis has an inner diameter of less than 0.2 millimetres – that is, the thickness of a piece of very fine cotton thread. The vas deferens is much thicker externally but it too is very narrow internally. If a blocked portion has to be removed and the tubing rejoined, the best results are obtained by microsurgery, with stitches so fine that they can hardly be seen at all with the naked eye. Although the surgery is technically difficult and a general anaesthetic is needed, recovery is very quick and there is hardly any pain so intercourse is not affected. A typical hospital stay is 2–4 days.

Results of microsurgery vary, depending on the position and extent of the block, and the expertise of the surgeon.[25] If the tubing has been blocked for a long time, the testicle tends gradually to stop producing sperm. Unfortunately, if production stops altogether, more sperm may not be made even when the tubing is unblocked. Eight per cent of infertile men have a block, and 20 to 30 per cent will produce normal sperm after this type of operation.

[25] This is very delicate surgery, requiring the steadiest hands. In order to avoid any hand tremor, some American surgeons claim they prepare for these operations for at least two days beforehand by not smoking, stopping all coffee, playing no tennis and avoiding sex. We don't in England. British surgeons believe that *thinking* about sex is what causes the tremor.

ASPIRATION OF THE EPIDIDYMIS

A very small number of infertile men, who have blockage of the vas deferens or epididymis, have been successfully treated by sucking sperms from the epididymal tubing using a fine needle. This is no small undertaking because it means a general anaesthetic, opening the testicle and puncturing the tubing. Most often no sperm are obtained, and those which are are immature and incapable of fertilisation. Moreover it does, of course, require IVF. Puncture of the epididymis is a procedure which can only be undertaken once or twice, because following this operation more scar tissue tends to develop in this extremely delicate tube. At the time of writing, only two babies have been born in Britain following this procedure.

ARTIFICIAL INSEMINATION WITH THE PARTNER'S SEMEN

Artificial insemination is the technique whereby sperm are injected into the woman by artificial means. It is most frequently performed using sperm from a donor – and this is discussed in detail in the next chapter. However, insemination with the male partner's semen, commonly known as 'artificial insemination by husband' (AIH), may be recommended in some cases when the sperm count is poor. Sperm can be inseminated by one of three well-tried methods.

INSEMINATION INTO THE CERVIX

Semen (usually produced by masturbation) is injected directly into the vagina through a small plastic tube so that it reaches the cervix. The woman has to lie on a couch with her knees up for about five minutes; the insemination itself causes no discomfort.

This kind of insemination is used for couples having difficulties with sexual intercourse; it may also be useful in the rare event of there being an anatomical problem with the uterus or cervix which prevents sperm finding the right place. Although this is controversial, I feel that there is usually little point in doing this if the man has a low sperm count because natural intercourse will achieve the same end: that is, introduction of sperm into the cervical canal. Although insemination causes no physical discomfort, the emotional pain may be considerable. One theoretical advantage of AIH is that insemination can be made at the most fertile moment – just before ovulation.

USING SPERM THAT HAVE BEEN SPECIALLY PROCESSED

The sperm are prepared after being produced by masturbation. They may be 'washed' – that is, the semen is repeatedly mixed with special laboratory fluid, i.e. medium, and the sperm are then removed by centrifugal force, by spinning the tube containing them. Alternatively, the sperm may be subjected to the 'swim' test (see p. 143). The semen is mixed with medium, healthy sperm are allowed to swim up to the surface under their own steam, and these are drawn off by suction through a glass tube. These healthy, concentrated sperm may then be inseminated into the cervix.

These methods may be used if there are large numbers of dead sperm or many dead cells in the semen. Strictly speaking, no real concentration of semen takes place, just a purification. These methods may also be used if there are sperm antibodies present, as the washing process may get rid of these.

Another method of preparing semen involves using a split ejaculate (see p. 145) to obtain the greater number of sperm that are present in the first part of the ejaculate. These would then be inseminated into the cervix. When used appropriately, these methods can result in pregnancy in around 30 per cent of subfertile couples, provided that the couple is prepared to persevere with several cycles of treatment.

INTRAUTERINE INSEMINATION

Occasionally doctors advise insemination directly into the uterus itself, bypassing the cervix. This is usually done when the woman has a cervical problem (*see* Chapter 6), but it is now being used for some cases of male infertility, especially when the sperm count is poor. Fresh, unwashed semen cannot be used because of a risk of infection and the sperm need to be prepared in the laboratory.

A fine tube containing sperm is inserted through the cervix and just into the uterus. This can cause minor discomfort, but there should be no pain. Early results are somewhat encouraging – a few doctors have had success with up to 35 per cent of couples, providing cycles are repeated for several months. There is evidence that the effect is improved slightly if the woman takes fertility drugs simultaneously, though it seems that the effect is only maintained if the drugs are given with regular ultrasound to the ovaries.

ARE THERE DISADVANTAGES TO INSEMINATION?

● The process itself tends to be very clinical and unspontaneous, and for some people this is almost worse than being infertile. There is no doubt that this treatment invades sex life to a greater extent than most doctors are prepared to admit or even realise.

● The man may not be able to masturbate to order. At the least, this will be embarrassing and, at worst, will cause feelings of guilt, frustration and anger. A great deal of patience and understanding are needed by both partners.

● Reasonably precise timing of ovulation is necessary. Temperature charting is insufficient, and the clinic should ask for blood tests, ultrasound or both. Regrettably, far too many clinics do not time this demanding treatment properly, so any benefit may be lost.

● Collecting a split ejaculate requires considerable manual dexterity right at the moment of orgasm.

● Sperm washing and the swim-up method require advanced laboratory facilities, and as the laboratory work is expensive and time-consuming, these are available only in relatively few centres.

● Insemination is unlikely to work in the first month. For the sperm to have a chance of being at the right place at the right moment, insemination may be done two or three times each month. Most couples who succeed with AIH do so only after several months. Many couples find AIH so frustrating and invasive of their sex lives that they give up after three or four months.

Treatment for the woman

FAILURE TO OVULATE

Treatment to restore ovulation is mostly successful. Unless the ovaries no longer have any eggs in them (premature menopause), modern drug therapy has at least an 80 per cent chance of producing regular ovulation. Unfortunately, for reasons that are not fully understood, probably only 65 per cent of women whose ovulation is successfully induced achieve pregnancy.

CLOMIPHENE

This is the commonly used fertility pill, normally marketed as Clomid or Serophene. Clomiphene is a very interesting compound. It was originally developed in an attempt to find a better contraceptive pill, one that did not have the side-effects associated with oestrogens. Clomiphene is technically an anti-oestrogen, with some of the properties of those hormones. When it was found that, when it was given to experimental rats, they still got pregnant, it was shelved. Some years later, a laboratory worker noted that the rats that had been given it were perhaps rather more fertile than average, and further tests were done. Eventually, in 1961, Dr Greenblatt and his colleagues working in the United States produced an epoch-making study of the value of clomiphene for women who fail to ovulate. Since then this drug has been responsible for more pregnancies in infertile patients than probably any other treatment in the world.

Clomiphene is an ideal, first-time treatment. It is cheap and free from major side-effects. It rarely causes multiple births because it is only a weak stimulant. It is thought to promote ovulation by stimulating the natural release of FSH from the pituitary. This makes the ovaries work harder and produce follicles.

In a way, clomiphene is a victim of its own success; it is too frequently given when it is not appropriate. Too many doctors prescribe it without making a diagnosis first. This has two drawbacks. First, it may delay finding the true cause for the infertility. Second, it can actually be contraceptive, which is why it was first developed. Because it is an anti-oestrogen, it can thicken cervical mucus, making the cervix unresponsive to sperm. It also appears to interfere with the uterine lining, which may prevent the early embryo implanting. These two points, plus the fact that occasionally clomiphene can make the ovaries cystic, are important reasons why this drug should only be taken when there is a genuine ovulation problem, and only under proper supervision.

How is clomiphene taken?

Usually, one tablet (50 mg) is taken every day for five days, starting from the first or second day of menstruation. If the cycle is much longer than twenty-eight days, clomiphene may be given from the fifth day for five days. The dose may be increased (two tablets daily, usually taken together) if there is no satisfactory response. There is no point in taking clomiphene for more than six days in each cycle, and doubling the dose beyond two tablets a day is seldom effective.

Unfortunately, clomiphene is unsuccessful in treating women over forty years old, especially when there is no clear evidence of ovulatory failure. In our practice, a live birth has happened only once.

How to know if the clomiphene is working

There may be symptoms which suggest ovulation – breast tenderness, mid-cycle discomfort in the abdomen, vaginal discharge near ovulation time, and/or painful and more regular periods. None of these, of course, proves ovulation. The doctor should check occasionally that ovulation is occurring, and the best way to do this is with ultrasound. This not only accurately confirms ovulation, but will also detect any cysts that might form. The alternative – a blood progesterone test – is commonly used but is far from reliable in this situation. This is because clomiphene can stimulate the ovary to produce more than one follicle simultaneously, none of which actually ovulates. The progesterone produced by all these follicles at once may raise blood levels of progesterone to an ovulatory value, even though an egg has not actually been shed.

What are the side-effects of clomiphene?

Clomiphene has few side-effects, and fewer risks. It can give hot flushes, the commonest problem. A few women notice increased abdominal discomfort at the time of ovulation; more likely, more painful periods are a sign that the drug is probably working. A few women get frequent or irregular periods – they generally should stop the drug. Any cysts which may very occasionally develop are not serious, but the drug should be stopped to give the ovary a chance to recover.

Some people wonder if clomiphene – or indeed any other drug designed to stimulate ovulation – could deplete the ovaries of eggs and cause a premature menopause. There is no evidence for this. Neither is there any truth in the idea that clomiphene can cause cancer of the ovary or uterus.

Unluckily, some people may just feel unwell while taking clomiphene. There are other, similar drugs that can be taken instead: tamoxifen (Tamofen) and cyclofenil (Rehibin). They frequently do not cause the unpleasant side-effects, but they are more expensive. They both can occasionally cause cysts, though.

How long should I take clomiphene?

This is very difficult to say. I personally cannot remember many women becoming pregnant if they have not conceived after nine ovulatory months on clomiphene. Of course, if clomiphene does not restore ovulation, it should be stopped sooner.

HUMAN CHORIONIC GONADOTROPHIN (HCG) INJECTIONS

HCG is similar in chemical structure to luteinising hormone (LH). Readers will recall that LH rises just before ovulation, triggering the release of the egg. HCG used to be prescribed with clomiphene; it was taken at mid-cycle to mimic the natural LH release so that the follicles, which have been stimulated by clomiphene, release the eggs they contain. There is now evidence that, unless injections are very carefully timed using blood tests and ultrasound, the HCG will have no useful effect. Indeed, given at the wrong time – say, more than 6–10 hours before or after – it might even interfere with the production of a fertilisable egg. This is why fewer doctors now recommend its use with clomiphene. It has very little or no value on its own.

BROMOCRIPTINE (PARLODEL)

These tablets are useful if the level of the hormone *prolactin* (*see* p. 146) is raised and there is no ovulation in consequence. Parlodel has also been prescribed in the past for unexplained infertility. This is now seldom done as there is no evidence that it is helpful unless there are high prolactin levels. If this really is the problem (and it is not very common), bromocriptine is a highly effective treatment.

It does have side-effects in some people. Apart from feeling rather unwell, they may feel faint or dizzy and occasionally nauseated. People should not drive a car during the first few days after starting bromocriptine; I have known one patient (in the early days of the use of this drug) who actually passed out twenty-four hours after starting this drug. Unfortunately, this happened while she was at the wheel of her car; luckily nobody was hurt. Of course, a complete faint is very unusual.

HUMAN MENOPAUSAL GONADOTROPHIN (HMG)

HMG (most commonly marketed as Pergonal or Humegon) is a mixture of the pituitary hormones LH and FSH, which stimulate the ovaries. Actually, the active ingredient is FSH; the LH content is not specially therapeutic in this context, but it is expensive to produce pure FSH. HMG is highly effective, but powerful and must be given under close supervision. Generally speaking, it is reserved for cases where clomiphene has failed. However, in certain women, it may be a first-line treatment, particularly if they are not having periods.

An important step in the research on human pituitary hormones was the recognition in 1960 that, during the menopause, the pituitary pours out large amounts of these hormones in an attempt by the body to stimulate the flagging ovaries. This excess LH and FSH spills over from the blood into the urine. In his original research Dr Donini in Rome processed 17,600 gallons of menopausal women's urine; Italy, of course, was a good source as there are large numbers of menopausal women living together in nunneries. This has been an excellent way of making HMG, but if you think about it, it is a bit ironic as this drug is now mainly used for IVF treatments, a therapy which is banned by the Roman Catholic Church.

HMG is given by injection from the early part of the menstrual cycle until ovulation is imminent – usually about five to ten days later. When ovulation is just about to occur, a triggering injection of human chorionic gonadotrophin (HCG) is given as, without this, the ovary will not usually shed the egg. This treatment is quite frequently used for women who are not having any periods at all. In this case, it is quite usual to stimulate a period first by giving the woman some progesterone pills.

Why women on HMG need careful monitoring

Treatment with HMG involves very careful control. It is usual to do daily ultrasound measurements of the follicles in the ovaries, and frequent assays of blood oestrogen are carried out by most clinics. There are two reasons why it is dangerous to take HMG without this close monitoring. First, some women overreact and their ovaries become very enlarged and cystic – the so-called *hyperstimulation syndrome*. Apart from being painful, this can be quite a serious condition and may require in-patient treatment in hospital. Second, because HMG frequently results in the ovary producing more than one follicle, each with its own egg, there is a serious risk of multiple ovulation. Indeed, nearly all the modern examples (much vaunted in the press) of serious multiple births – that is, triplets, quadruplets and quin-tuplets – have occurred after this treatment. Monitoring helps avoid this problem. If too many follicles are seen on ultrasound, the triggering dose of HCG can be withheld.

The possibility of triplets may seem wonderful for people who have been persistently infertile for years. It is not. Multiple pregnancy is much more tiring and dangerous for the mother, carries a serious risk of miscarriage, stillbirth and early loss of the babies and presents couples with great difficulties in the first year or two after birth. Any pregnancy involving more than twins is best avoided if at all possible. Fortunately, with proper care, these complications do not occur.

How long is it worth trying treatment with HMG?

HMG is an expensive drug, and the proper monitoring for it complex. We find that it costs at least £180 for one month's supply of the drug, and because we believe in very careful monitoring, we probably spend at least another £150 in monitoring each cycle. The total cost in a well-run unit, then, is likely to be more than £350 per month. Consequently, most clinics offer treatment for only three months at a time. At the end of that period, the treatment needs careful review. Frankly, if conception has not happened after definite ovulation in each of six cycles with HMG, there is less than a 10 per cent chance with continued treatment.

PUMP THERAPY

In a normal person, both FSH and LH are released from the pituitary gland in pulses. There is not a steady stream of production, but rather intermittent bursts occur at intervals of every 60–90 minutes. Why this is so is not understood. However, it is thought by some that, as these gonadotrophins are naturally produced in this way, it would be more physiological to inject HMG in similar pulses.

To save the poor patient an injection every hour, she wears a little battery-operated electric pump attached to a syringe. This can easily be strapped to an arm, and is soon forgotten. Every ninety minutes or so (the interval can be varied), the little pump does its work and a small amount of hormone painlessly enters the bloodstream. There is an impression that pump therapy may help ovulation, particularly in some cases of polycystic ovary disease.

PURE FSH TREATMENT

During the past few years, pure FSH has been available. Initially, there was great excitement about it as it was widely expected to be much more effective than HMG. In fact, pure FSH (brand name Metrodin) has proved to be a disappointment. It is as good as HMG, but no better except in certain specific and unusual cases. We have had some success with a special low-dose régime with this drug; this is not as expensive and may have a place for women with polycystic ovaries.

GENETICALLY ENGINEERED FSH

Two major drug companies have wanted to get out of nuns' urine for some years. Biologically derived drugs do have certain problems, the possibility of contamination and the difficulty of standardising the effectiveness of the drug being two of them.

Modern genetic methods meant that the gene responsible for the production of FSH by the human pituitary could be identified and manufactured. This gene has been successfully artificially incorporated into the Chinese Hamster ovary. Genetically engineered isolated cells, taken from hamster ovaries, are placed in a massive vat in a kind of soup which is kept under rigid conditions. This avoids the problems with drugs taken from human sources, such as urine. The pure FSH which is produced is very potent and is likely eventually to provide very much better fertility treatments with more precise and powerful stimulation of the ovaries. At the time of writing, we are using this drug in human patients on an experimental basis. The results are encouraging. Unfortunately, one problem is that these drugs have been very expensive to research and produce.[26]

TREATMENT WITH RELEASING HORMONE (LHRH)

The normal production of the pituitary hormones LH and FSH depends on the secretion of releasing hormones from the hypothalamus in the brain. Just as LH and FSH are produced in pulses, so is the stimulus from the hypothalamus. In 1979 it was shown that the injection of LH-releasing hormone (usually called LHRH) in regular pulses could produce ovulation. This treatment is particularly useful when the communication between the hypothalamus and pituitary gland is not working normally. It involves the woman wearing a pump (like the pump therapy described above), which injects the required amount of releasing hormone at regular intervals.

LHRH therapy has less risk of producing a multiple pregnancy than does treatment with pituitary hormones. This is because the pituitary is left to work on its own and can regulate its activity depending on how much hormone the ovaries actually need.

---

[26] This cost, of course, will be borne by the consumer. Drug companies are currently very coy about how much this treatment is likely to cost, and I have doubts that the benefits will be sufficiently great to justify the extra expense.

DRUGS WHICH STOP THE PITUITARY GLAND
FROM WORKING

In the last few years, there has been a significant breakthrough with drugs which 'freeze' the pituitary gland. The discovery and synthesis of LHRH led to the development of compounds that are chemically similar and which have powerful medical applications. The one most commonly used to treat infertility is buserelin (Suprefact).

Buserelin currently comes in the form of a nasal spray. Because it is short-acting, it needs to be taken every four hours, and last thing at night and first thing in the morning. There are other, longer-acting drugs being developed which will be less inconvenient, but so far there has not been adequate time to prove their safety. When buserelin is first given, it stimulates the pituitary to produce more FSH and LH. This effect only lasts a day or two, following which the production of these two hormones falls dramatically and stays low. Long-term (more than a few days) administration of buserelin therefore results in the ovaries becoming inactive, no longer stimulated by the pituitary hormones. Oestrogen production falls to low levels. In effect, a woman taking buserelin becomes menopausal – a very strange treatment, seemingly, for somebody wanting to get pregnant.

However, once buserelin has suppressed the ovaries, they are very receptive to gonadotrophins such as HMG, given by injection. The latest research shows that sometimes the eggs which are produced by this method are of 'better quality' and more likely to produce a successfully growing embryo. Moreover, the ovaries seem able to produce more eggs simultaneously when buserelin is used, and this may be of particular benefit during IVF treatment (see p. 203).

Buserelin treatment with HMG is now being used for women who respond poorly to HMG alone and not at all to clomiphene. It probably is most suitable for those who have polycystic ovaries. If this is the problem, it may be well worth while asking the specialist more about it.

PROGESTERONES

Some women are said to have a 'deficient luteal phase' when the ovary does not produce enough progesterone after ovulation. It is claimed (though there are many arguments against this) that this leads to the endometrium being underdeveloped and incapable of receiving a fertilised egg satisfactorily. Some doctors give progesterone, usually by injection or by a vaginal pessary, in the hope of a better environment development inside the uterus. Others give injections of HCG which stimulates the ovaries to produce their own progesterone after ovulation. There is very little evidence that these treatments work.

SURGICAL WEDGE RESECTION OF THE OVARIES

Many years ago, before the powerful drugs that stimulate ovulation were developed, it was discovered that removing a piece of the ovary surgically could actually help ovulation, and that this treatment worked particularly well in some forms of polycystic ovary syndrome. It used to be thought that the effect was produced by breaking the thick ovarian capsule, which subsequently allowed the trapped eggs to escape. However, this operation fell into disrepute, partly because it involved opening the abdomen and partly because it tended to cause adhesion formation, which could prevent the tubes from functioning properly.

There has, however, been a recent revival of interest in this operation, for two reasons. First, by using microsurgery or a laparoscope the risk of adhesion formation has been abolished. Second, it has been found to be effective in some women when all drug treatment has repeatedly failed. It now is thought to work possibly by altering the powerful growth factors in the ovary, which can change the growth of the follicles. Seven of our patients have become pregnant after this operation in the last two years. A recently developed alternative is gently to drill the ovarian capsule by burning it at laparoscopy, which is simpler and probably as effective.

Rarely, a very raised prolactin level may mean a benign tumour of the pituitary. Most of these respond to drug treatment alone, using bromocriptine. Occasionally, however, the tumour may be too large for this and, if left untreated, could affect eyesight. A hospital CAT scan may be requested. This is a special computerised X-ray, which will give information about the size and position of the tumour. If it is very large, the doctor may advise surgery. Rest assured, this kind of pituitary surgery is not life-threatening. It generally results in a woman not producing enough pituitary hormones, but these can be replaced by drugs. I have seen many successful pregnancies following this surgery and treatment with hormones.

TUBAL DAMAGE AND ADHESIONS IN THE ABDOMEN

Treatments for disease of the Fallopian tubes, or for adhesions in and around the tubes and ovaries, involve some form of surgery. Until about 1970, tubal surgery was well known to have abysmal results. A survey of the world literature showed that, if the tubes were completely blocked, no more than 10 per cent of women had a live baby following surgery. Even when the tubes were damaged but not blocked, surgery to release adhesions (when internal organs have become stuck together) gave, at best, no more than about a 25 per cent chance of a live baby afterwards. Naturally, this dismal record greatly influenced many infertility specialists. Many gave up surgery completely. Others invariably advised women to avoid having tubal damage corrected. Tubal surgery was left to a handful of enthusiasts, who continued to do their best.

The internal diameter of the human Fallopian tube is very fine. At the tube's narrowest point the fertilised egg goes through a tunnel less than 0.4 millimetres in diameter – the thickness of a piece of thick thread. Hardly surprising, then, that operations to join up this portion of the tube, performed with the naked eye alone, were so unsuccessful. It was only when operating microscopes became widely available and were adapted for abdominal surgery in the 1970s that tubal surgery became a viable option for women with blocked tubes. Within a few years, success rates were doubled, trebled or even quadrupled in some cases. Regrettably, in the United Kingdom, where the treatment was pioneered, microsurgery has been slow to be properly implemented. Consequently, some women still get operations which fall well short of the ideal.

WHAT IS TUBAL MICROSURGERY?

Microsurgery is any form of surgery involving the use of a microscope and very fine instruments. Nearly all patients with pelvic adhesions or damage inside the abdomen causing infertility also have some damage to their tubes, hence the word 'tubal'. Tubal microsurgery is a term which is loosely used to include not only operations on the Fallopian tubes but also those on the ovaries, or even sometimes the uterus. In my view, virtually all operations in a woman's pelvis should involve the use of a microscope. These tissues are extremely delicate and easily damaged. Adhesion formation, which can make some severely infertile, is very common after operations using conventional methods and not the specialised equipment which is essential for the best results. Unfortunately, once a woman has developed adhesions following naked-eye surgery, adhesions can be extremely difficult or even impossible to treat.

The following are the most important and frequently performed operations:

DIVISION OF ADHESIONS

The most common operation is division of adhesions around the tubes, ovaries or the uterus. The technical term is *adhesiolysis*, or *salpingolysis* if the tubes are involved. These operations do not always need a microscope, but the surgeon should always employ some form of magnification, perhaps with magnifying spectacles. Success rates average between 30 and 65 per cent, depending on the extent of adhesions. The success rate when magnification is not used is less than half that obtained following microsurgery.

OPENING THE OVARIAN END OF THE TUBES

Most tubal blockage involves the delicate outer end of the tube, the *fimbria*, which are near the ovary and which pick up the egg. When this end of the tube is blocked, fluid fills the tube and a swelling called a *hydrosalpinx* forms. The operation to open the tube is known as a *salpingostomy*. The success of this depends on:

1. the degree of damage;
2. whether a microscope is used.

The scientific literature shows that when the naked eye is employed for salpingostomy only 8 per cent of patients later conceive; with the microscope, up to 40 per cent of them do.

If the tubes are fibrous (thickened with scar tissue) or the tubal lining is very flattened and damaged (usually diagnosed with a careful X-ray), tubal surgery of any kind will give very poor results and we prefer to offer IVF. About 8 per cent of all pregnancies after salpingostomy (including those resulting from IVF treatment) end as ectopic pregnancies (*see* Chapter 13).

OPENING THE UTERINE END OF THE TUBES

This is one of the great success stories of modern infertility treatment. Until the microscope was employed for this operation in 1975, the standard operation was *tubal implantation*, in which the blocked part of the tube was removed and the remainder of the tube was implanted in the uterus through a new hole bored into its wall. Only 20 per cent of the patients conceived, but after microsurgery between 45 to 65 per cent of women have a live baby.

The modern operation is called *cornual anastomosis*, in which the blocked part of the tube is removed and the remainder is stitched back on to the original opening. It is difficult technically and fairly time-consuming, but the surgical effort is certainly worth it, particularly as the ectopic pregnancy rate afterwards is only about 3 per cent.

REVERSAL OF STERILISATION

A few women bitterly regret their decision to be sterilised. Women who are unfortunate to be in this position will hopefully recall that the decision was, in all probability, taken at a moment of great stress and pressure, or at least when their circumstances were substantially different. Microsurgery has been highly successful in reconstituting tubes which have been previously cut or tied.[27] If sterilisation has been done with a clip (a frequently used method), reversal is very like to be possible. Overall, success rates vary from between 65 per cent and 95 per cent, largely depending on the experience of the surgeon, whether a microscope is used, and the type of sterilisation being reversed. However, surgery is not a satisfactory option if nearly all of both tubes have been badly damaged or removed.

WHAT DOES THIS SURGERY INVOLVE?

Tubal microsurgery tends to take a bit longer than conventional surgery – in skilled hands no more than an extra thirty or forty minutes – but nobody feels worse after surgery because of this. On the contrary, because this surgery is done with delicacy, most patients recover far quicker than after conventional pro-

[27] Fifteen years ago, when this surgery was very new, I was invited to demonstrate this approach in Los Angeles, California. I was joined by Victor Gomel, the well-known infertility surgeon from Vancouver, Canada. We operated in an amazing new operating threatre on closed-circuit television, and the picture was beamed to a lecture hall some five miles away, where 600 surgeons watched. We had no chance to select the patient, a woman sterilised at twenty-one years old, weighing twenty-two stone. Victor did the left tube, I repaired the right. We struggled for five hours to complete this dreadful procedure with the wrong instruments, an inadequate microscope, an unhelpful theatre staff and, forgetting we were being broadcast, some choice four-letter words. People said afterwards it was the most entertaining TV programme they had ever watched. When this lady surprisingly got pregnant some months later, I often wondered whether conception occurred through Victor's side, or mine.

cedures. Nearly all surgeons now use a 'bikini' incision – that is, a cut in the skin which goes across the pubic-hair line, and which leaves only a very faint scar after six months. Most of my own patients usually remain in hospital for about five days afterwards, but different hospitals may have different routines. There is some discomfort, but never unbearable pain. The most common problem is 'wind', with swelling of the abdomen which can be very uncomfortable for about two days afterwards.

WHAT HAPPENS AFTER TUBAL MICROSURGERY?

The first major event, which so many people worry about quite needlessly is removal of stitches, usually done on the seventh day after the operation. This takes only a few seconds and is painless; surprising how many people panic.

The real path to recovery takes place after stitch removal. Obviously, the way individuals tolerate surgery varies. Some find that they are ready to go back to even quite energetic work within two weeks of leaving hospital. Equally, others may take much longer to recover fully. It is very usual to find oneself more tired than normal for at least four or five weeks after tubal surgery.

At first, it is reasonable not to strain the abdomen. There is no need to worry too much about this; the importance of not carrying heavy weights is exaggerated. It is wise not to strain oneself too much for the first two weeks after leaving hospital because this can delay wound healing and make the abdomen very sore. Coughing, or straining on going to the toilet, may cause apprehension (or soreness) but no serious problems. It is impossible to damage the tubes themselves, no matter how much one strains.

SEX AFTER SURGERY

Basically, there is no harm in having sex as soon as both partners feel like it. The operation cannot be damaged, nor the tubes blocked. It may simply be the last thing on anybody's mind when they leave hospital, though things may feel very different 12–14 days later.

> The unofficial world record for post-surgical sex is, as far as I know, held by a twenty-seven-year-old American. I operated on Jane on a Wednesday, opening both tubes in a two-hour operation, through quite a large hole in her abdomen. Late the following sultry Saturday afternoon, seventy-five hours after waking from anaesthesia, the ward nurse, a rather shy girl, was doing her rounds. Entering Jane's side-ward, she saw our patient and her large Texan partner in an extremely interesting position. Nursing manuals do not give much advice about what to do in situations like this. Jane had a positive pregnancy test sixteen days later. A letter she sent me recently tells me that her little boy is exceptionally good at sport.
>
> The British record would appear to be held by Anne, a very pretty Welsh lady. She only had one remaining tube which was totally blocked, the other having been removed some years earlier. She was advised by a private clinic that in vitro fertilisation would be a much better treatment than tubal surgery. After in vitro fertilisation had failed twice, she was referred to my clinic. I suggested we opened her remaining tube surgically. She, at least, had the decency to wait after her operation until the evening after her skin stitches were removed, six days after surgery. She conceived, and at the time of writing, the pregnancy is progressing well.

SEEING THE DOCTOR AFTER MICROSURGERY

Regular clinic attendance is, I think, essential after tubal surgery. We like to see all our patients every three months until they get pregnant, or until they decide to give up or to try alternative treatments. This allows us to do a good deal of fine tuning, such as rechecking ovulation, the sperm counts and generally ensuring that fertility is maximised.

If there are any gynaecological symptoms after surgery, I

strongly advise an appointment to see the doctor promptly. It is possible to get further inflammation or infection, and this needs the promptest treatment. People who think they may be pregnant, by even a few days, should seek medical advice. There is a somewhat higher risk of ectopic pregnancy once the tubes have been cleared after surgery (*see* Chapter 13), and the specialist may suggest an ultrasound examination and routine blood tests to exclude this.

If there is still no pregnancy after a year of trying, a laparoscopic examination may be very worth while. This will confirm whether or not the tubes are still in good condition, and whether or not there are any adhesions. Some clinics do an X-ray but this does not give nearly as much information, and risks more inflammation. Those who are older than average – say, more than thirty-six – may consider having a laparoscopy earlier than one year after surgery, so that they can decide whether or not to enter an in vitro fertilisation programme.

FEELINGS AFTER TUBAL SURGERY

Women vary in how they feel after tubal surgery. Some feel much more optimistic and, if they don't get pregnant, come to terms with it. Others, especially if they have not been carefully advised beforehand, expect to get pregnant immediately and feel increasingly let down and anxious when they have a period each month. Tubal surgery does not often work immediately, and unless women, especially, remember this, they may end each month feeling quite devastated at the start of a period, particularly if this happens a day or two late. Following any fertility surgery, there is a 10 per cent chance of conception each month at best. It is essential, therefore, to get things in perspective.

Emma is a well-to-do housewife. Both her tubes had become blocked near the uterus following an infection after a miscarriage. I performed cornual anastomosis surgery when she was thirty-four. She was very depressed when she did not conceive immediately, even though I felt the operation had gone really well. Within three months of surgery, she became increasingly concerned and tearful and asked to be treated by in vitro fertilisation. At that time, IVF was even more unsuccessful than it is now, and I refused her as gently as I could. She immediately referred herself to another unit, and over the next two years had four unsuccessful treatments with IVF, never really giving herself a chance to come to terms with her problem. She then returned to our clinic and had extensive counselling and joined our support group. Three years after the operation, she had her first baby, James; since then she has had another boy and, ten months ago, a baby girl.

WHAT ABOUT THE LASER TO UNBLOCK TUBES?

There has been a huge amount of publicity about the use of lasers in surgery generally, and for infertile patients particularly. Many advantages are claimed for tubal microsurgery using lasers, including less blood loss, more accuracy in cutting, greater speed and less adhesion formation. In fact, the only advantage that is not claimed for laser microsurgery is that there is a better chance of pregnancy if the laser is used.

My own bias is that the laser is not useful for any tubal surgery when the abdomen is opened. I actually find the surgery takes me longer with a laser, and that healing is no better than the fine microsurgery with diathermy (when blood vessels are sealed with the heat from a high-frequency electric current); consequently, we stopped using the laser some time ago. Certainly lasers are very useful for the treatment of pre-cancer of the cervix, where a cervical smear may be abnormal. However, there is no evidence that the chances of pregnancy occurring are higher with laser, and this lack of evidence, rather than the expense involved, has persuaded the National Health Service in the UK that extra lasers are not needed. Perhaps the only justification for the use of lasers in tubal surgery is during laparoscopy (*see* below), and this is doubtful.

SURGERY DONE DOWN THE LAPAROSCOPE

In recent years, there has been considerable interest in surgery done during a laparoscopy. The laparoscope is introduced in the usual way, through a small hole in the navel. One or two small cuts about one inch in length (2.5 cm) are made in the abdomen low down near the pubic-hair line and fine instruments are introduced through these holes. Long fine scissors or tweezers can be introduced and adhesions cut. Some surgeons even feel confident enough to open the ends of the tubes, if they are blocked near ovaries. Cutting has to be done with some care, and all blood is continuously washed off the tissues using a fine jet of fluid also introduced through the abdominal wall. This can then be sucked out with a small tube. Bleeding can be controlled using a special diathermy machine.

Some surgeons use a laser beam as their main instrument during laparoscopic surgery. They claim that this gives better control over bleeding, which is probably true. Whether the cutting is more accurate I rather doubt. The main advantage with laparoscopic surgery, whether done with a laser or not, is the rapidity with which women recover. Usually only a single overnight stay in hospital is required, and there is no abdominal wound which takes time to heal. Results are best in experienced surgical hands.

The success rates with this kind of surgery are claimed to be high, but they do not seem to be as good as those after open microsurgery. Unfortunately, laparoscopic surgery is not always possible.

PASSING BALLOONS OR DILATORS INTO THE TUBE

Some doctors have recently begun to use fine dilators (or balloons), which are passed through the uterus into the tube, to treat blockages where the tube joins the uterus. It requires the use of X-rays to guide the surgeon, and can be done without an anaesthetic. It is similar to the recent invention of angioplasty, when radiologists pass thin tubes into blood vessels in the heart to widen them and prevent angina and heart attacks. It may have an application in fertility surgery – certainly it saves hospital admission – but there is, as yet, little evidence of its value since there have been few pregnancies.

TREATING ENDOMETRIOSIS

Treatment for endometriosis (see p. 107) is a very controversial issue. Some doctors feel that endometriosis never causes infertility, except when it causes severe distortion and scarring of the tissues, or when it results in bad adhesions around the tubes and ovaries. Others believe that even mild endometriosis should be treated, because it may cause infertility, and it may get worse and cause bad scarring and distortion, with tubal and ovarian damage. I personally am in the 'no treatment' camp, except when there is clearly severe distortion, or if a woman is suffering pain or discomfort – a common symptom.

LAPAROSCOPIC SURGERY WITH OR WITHOUT THE LASER

Spots of endometriosis can be burned with diathermy or laser, during a laparoscopy. The advantages are that it can be done at the time a diagnosis is made, it does not require major surgery and, unlike drug treatment, it does not stop ovulation. However, there are a number of disadvantages: it is expensive, and not always available; it must be performed while under a general anaesthetic; and there is absolutely no evidence that one is more likely to conceive afterwards.

DRUG TREATMENT

Drug treatments depend for their effect on the fact that endometriosis, like the endometrium (womb lining), is hormone-dependent, that is, it grows when there is enough oestrogen around. Therefore, the aim of all drug treatment is to reduce the amount of oestrogen in the body and thus cause the endometriosis to stop spreading and perhaps shrink.

The most widely used drugs are probably the contraceptive

pill and progesterone-like drugs. They damp down ovarian activity and the endometriosis melts away. Another commonly used drug is danazol (Danol), which is a compound that resembles testosterone (male hormone) and which also markedly reduces ovarian activity. A third group of drugs, recently introduced, are the LHRH analogues (buserelin is one example; see p. 175). These produce a temporary menopause, and the endometriosis shrinks away.

The advantages of drug treatment for endometriosis are that no surgery is needed, any pain is always improved and it may prevent the spread of endometriosis. However, some women feel very unwell on these drugs. Moreover conception is almost impossible while taking such drugs and endometriosis tends to regrow as soon as they are stopped.

MICROSURGERY

One reasonably effective way of dealing with endometriosis is to remove it surgically, and it may be the best way of stopping its recurrence. When endometriosis is very extensive, it is often not feasible to remove all the affected tissue; neither is the use of a microscope particularly helpful. Conversely, open surgery is not justified if the disease is mild.

With microsurgery, one can try to get pregnant immediately one recovers. In addition, it is the only reliable way of treating endometriosis that is causing cysts on the ovary, and it is the best chance to prevent a recurrence of the disease. On the other hand, it does involve an operation and being out of action for about three weeks.

All treatments for endometriosis carry about a 60 per cent change of pregnancy at best. If the endometriosis is extensive, the success rate will be considerably less. Ocassionaly I get the strong feeling that women become pregnant in spite of the treatment: certainly if mild endometriosis is left untreated, the chances of pregnancy are as good as if it is treated.

IN VITRO FERTILISATION OR GIFT

This may be justified when endometriosis is causing infertility (*see* Chapter 11).

PROBLEMS IN THE UTERUS

Uterine problems may require a surgical approach. Many of these operations are relatively minor, and can be done on an out-patient basis. A few are occasionally treatable with drugs.

FIBROIDS

Fibroids (*see* p. 89) can certainly cause infertility if they are close to the uterine cavity and distort it, or if they displace the ovaries, or if they grow close to where the Fallopian tube enters the uterus, causing a blockage. Treatment is generally surgical. The operation to remove fibroids is called *myomectomy* and is fairly similar to tubal microsurgery. The fibroids are removed from the uterus, usually after cutting into the uterine muscle. It is rather like cutting cleanly into a peach to remove the stone, without disturbing the flesh of the peach too much. Following removal of the fibroid, the space where it lay is carefully stitched together, and the muscle of the uterus is also repaired with stitches.

The uterus has a fairly good blood supply and may bleed during the procedure. This is why it is usual to make sure that some blood of the right blood group is on hand in case the bleeding is vigorous. This is just for safety's sake – in practice, a blood transfusion is very rarely needed.

When this operation is done in women under the age of thirty-five, about 65 per cent will conceive. It is much less successful after this age, with only about 35 per cent becoming pregnant.

CONGENITAL ABNORMALITIES

Perhaps the most important of these is a *septate uterus* (*see* pp. 109–10). This can usually be dealt with by simply cutting it using an hysteroscope (telescope inside the uterus). This is a very effective treatment and can usually be done with no more than an overnight stay in hospital. There may be a little vaginal bleeding afterwards, but usually no more than during a period. If the septum is very large, the doctor may prefer to remove it by opening the uterus from above and performing an operation rather like removal of a fibroid. The chance of pregnancy afterwards is about 75 per cent.

An uncommon abnormality is a *double uterus*. This may be repaired by joining the two halves of the uterus together. This kind of surgery is rather specialised and is best done in a centre where a good deal of this work goes on. Unfortunately, if the operation goes badly, it can't easily be changed later. Properly done uterine reconstruction of this sort (called *utriculoplasty*) carries a 65 per cent chance of pregnancy.

The third abnormality is a *rudimentary uterine horn*. This is usually the less well-formed half of a double uterus. It may justify open surgery.

INTERNAL ADHESIONS (SYNECHIAE)

These cause the walls of the uterus to stick together and can usually be separated by a simple vaginal operation. The surgeon may use a hysteroscope and special scissors or a laser. The operation can be done as a day-case, under quick anaesthesia, and may need repeating. Some patients have needed five of these little operations spaced over several months. Sometimes it is necessary to place a plastic coil (an IUD) in the uterus for a few weeks afterwards to keep the uterine walls apart. Antibiotics may also be given, and sometimes steroid and oestrogen tablets, all of which help healing. The chance of a pregnancy after this operation is about 70 per cent.

POLYPS

Nowadays, this is really about the only serious indication for an infertile woman to have a D & C (dilatation of the cervix and curettage), or 'scrape'. Removal of a large polyp – which is not very common – gives a good chance of pregnancy on the rare occasions when it is the cause of the infertility.

ADENOMYOSIS

This puzzling condition, where the uterus becomes increasingly scarred following invasion of its muscle with lining tissue, is very difficult to treat. As we have seen with endometriosis (*see* above) the endometrium (or lining tissue) is sensitive to the ovarian hormone oestrogen. If the level of this in the body is reduced, the lining tissue is reduced as well. The usual treatment, therefore, is the same as drug treatment for endometriosis. This damps down hormones and will control painful or irregular periods, but it will not help getting pregnant. Surgery will not help either. Generally it is impossible to remove the adenomyosis without damage to the uterus. Fortunately only a few women become infertile as a result of it. Women with adenomyosis have about a 35 per cent chance of getting pregnant.

PROBLEMS WITH THE CERVICAL MUCUS

Just how important cervical mucus problems are is difficult to say. There is probably as much nonsense written about cervical mucus as there is about any other topic in infertility. We have tried various treatments to improve the numbers of sperm to the cervical mucus. Sometimes we find that the test becomes positive and, within a few cycles, there is a pregnancy. There is no evidence that these women would not have got pregnant without treatment.

DOUCHING WITH BICARBONATE OF SODA

Many women are advised to douche with a weak alkali, such as bicarbonate of soda, to soften the mucus and to correct acidity. The belief is that the sperm are being killed by acid vaginal secretions but this is fallacious as all women normally have an acid vagina, nature's protection against infection. Moreover, the sperm stay in the cervical canal inside the mucus, which is not acid and which is generally not affected by the vaginal fluid. There is no evidence that any form of douche improves a woman's fertility.

In 1988, that highly respectable professional publication, the *British Journal of Obstetrics and Gynaecology* reported a curious example of how acid does not always kill the sperm. It told of a young lady from South Africa born with a rare abnormality – a completely absent vagina. This causes complete sterility, because the uterus has no communication with the outside world. One evening she was satisfying the desires of a friend by indulging him with oral sex. At a rather crucial moment, an ex-boyfriend rushed into her bedroom and glimpsing the proceedings, seized a knife, stabbing her in the abdomen, piercing her stomach. She was rushed to hospital, in mortal danger from the resulting injury.

During the subsequent emergency operation to save her life, surgeons washed out her stomach and abdominal cavity which was of course, filled with the natural, very acid secretions which the stomach produces. Nine months later, she was delivered of a live baby by Caesarean section, there being no other outlet for the baby. Sperm had survived the highly concentrated acid in the stomach and clearly must have been washed into the Fallopian tubes, where they successfully fertilised an egg.

OESTROGEN TABLETS AND VAGINAL CREAMS

Oestrogens help the cervix to produce great quantities of watery mucus. This does seem to improve the post-coital test in some people, and pregnancies are reported, but we do not know whether the apparent improvements in cervical mucus are the real cause of these pregnancies. Taking oestrogen in small doses (even by a cream in the vagina) can help some women ovulate, and it could just be that the pregnancies which seem to occur with oestrogen therapy happen because of improved ovulation rather than improved mucus.

STEROID TABLETS

Cortisone-like drugs may be given if there are antibodies attacking the sperm as they enter the mucus. Although there is some evidence that this may be of benefit, my own feeling is that it is not really safe for a woman to take steroids for this purpose. A short course of two or three weeks at a time might be reasonable, but long-term steroid treatment can cause stomach ulcers, changes in the bones with loss of calcium, emotional disturbances and increased susceptibility to infection. Steroids are probably best reserved for life-threatening diseases.

CRYOTHERAPY OR LASER TREATMENT

One theory is that abnormal (sperm-resistant) mucus is made by abnormal cervical gland cells, and if these are frozen, or burned, normal surface gland cells will tend to grow in their place, and this will possibly promote the production of good mucus. At least these treatments are painless and cause little inconvenience. They can be done during a simple visit to the clinic.

ANTIBIOTIC TREATMENT

It has been said that one reason why the cervix may not let the sperm survive is because of infection. Various bugs have been incriminated. It has been fashionable to blame Chlamydia, mycoplasmas and ureaplasmas, partly because these ill-understood bacteria are often found on the cervix. Unfortunately for the pundits, these bacteria may also linger in the cervix and vagina of normally fertile women. Some years ago, a very clever study was done which showed that whether one had treatment for these bacteria or not made absolutely no difference to fertility. In fact, women who were not treated actually got pregnant faster. This has not stopped many doctors from continuing to give women drugs against these infections.

More importantly, many women who are infertile worry greatly that a thrush infection or an infection with trichomonas, both of which are very common in the vagina, is preventing them from getting pregnant. This worry is quite without foundation, unless of course symptoms from the infection (such as soreness) are preventing them from having intercourse.

ARTITICIAL INSEMINATION WITH THE PARTNER'S SPERM

Generally speaking, there is usually little point in artificial insemination with one's partner's sperm (AIH). This bypasses the cervix by putting sperm directly into the uterus, but there is very little evidence that it will do much good. My feeling is that a man can do that perfectly well himself and usually with much greater pleasure for both partners.

There is a very important point here. Repeated post-coital tests and inseminations may well be more than either partner may feel like bearing. Most people find it very unpleasant to have sex 'to order', and regular attendances to have insemination by a white-coated doctor can greatly interfere with one's self-esteem and one's sex life. All of us repeatedly see women conceive without any treatment, in spite of many negative post-coital tests.

CHAPTER TEN

Unexplained Infertility

The label 'unexplained infertility' is a good example of medical failure. Whilst this is controversial, it seems extremely unsatisfactory to 'diagnose' a couple as suffering from 'unexplained infertility'. Some textbooks and articles even give it a name – 'idiopathic infertility' – as if this makes it respectable. Of course, all that 'idiopathic' means is 'unexplained'. Doctors, like most other professionals, are relieved to shelter behind a long, complicated word, if the confusion it causes in others hides their own confusion. Some clinics even state that as many as 25–30 per cent of their patients suffer from unexplained infertility. My own view is that, if the doctor looks hard enough, a clear cause for the infertility can usually be found. This may mean doing very careful tests, and sometimes even repeating tests. At Hammersmith, we calculate that only 5 per cent of our patients have truly unexplained infertility.

Why does all this matter? There are basically three reasons:
● First, when the cause for the infertility is not available, treatment cannot be rational. Various 'remedies' will be tried on a purely haphazard basis. Consequently, luck will play a greater part in whether or not the woman gets pregnant.
● Second, there will be inevitable pressure to turn to the 'high tech' treatments, particularly IVF or GIFT, in the hope of striking lucky. This involves the couple in complex and demanding medicine, which may delay a correct diagnosis and more effective treatment being commenced.
● Third, infertility is emotionally taxing. It is very much easier to come to terms with infertility, even if one never

conceives, if it is possible to find out what has been causing it. A 'diagnosis' of unexplained infertility throws an extra psychological burden on a couple.

What are the likely causes of 'unexplained' infertility?

Some years ago, we completed a survey of patients who had been told at some time that they had unexplained infertility. All had been infertile for a minimum of three years. Some had been trying for a baby as long as seventeen years; all of them had seen at least one specialist and had been advised to try a 'high tech' treatment such as IVF.

Each of these couples was carefully reinvestigated. The preliminary results make interesting reading because, in about 80 per cent of cases, we felt we could identify a clearly treatable cause for the infertility. Many of these couples with a newly identified cause for their infertility have now undergone quite simple, but specific, treatments of various kinds in our clinic and already more than one-third of the women are pregnant or have delivered, without recourse to IVF. The following are the most common problems we found.

● *An unexpected problem in the man*. Although all the men had initially had normal sperm counts, when the sperm were subjected to a separation test (*see* p. 143), we discovered that many semen specimens showed subtle but important abnormalities. Moreover, we confirmed that, when the separation test improved, a pregnancy often occurred soon afterwards, frequently within two or three months. Sometimes semen from apparently normal men in partnerships with unexplained infertility simply fails to fertilise eggs when IVF is eventually undertaken. It may be some years before we fully understand this defect. Conclusion: at least 30 per cent of unexplained infertility is due to poor sperm function.

● *A problem in the uterus*. Many women with unexplained infertility had not had the uterus properly evaluated. A majority had not had an X-ray (hysterosalpingogram); in other cases, the X-ray which had been done was not of sufficient quality to make a proper diagnosis. On careful re-evaluation, we found a high proportion of women had adhesions, fibroids, or polyps in the cavity of the uterus, or adenomyosis. Approximately half of those treated for fibroids, polyps or adhesions conceived; adenomyosis treatment gave very poor results. Conclusion: about 20 per cent of unexplained infertility is due to a significant uterine problem.

● *Subtle problems with ovulation.* Many women turned out not to be ovulating every month, or to be ovulating but with subtle problems making their hormones abnormal. Recent evidence suggests that ovulating women with hormonal problems may be quite infertile and that correction of the hormone problem is well worth while. Several of the women we examined with ultrasound had polycystic ovaries, but it is less clear whether this was causing the infertility. Some women had a poor response to drugs given to stimulate ovulation when treated by IVF. Very often, inadequate blood tests for hormone levels had been done during IVF so the fault was not immediately obvious and left uncorrected. Conclusion: at least 15 per cent of unexplained infertility is associated with abnormal hormone secretion, which affects ovulation, the quality of eggs, or uterine environment.

● *Tubal problems and endometriosis.* A surprising number of women had some degree of tubal damage, which showed up on a careful repeat laparoscopy or hysterosalpingogram. In some cases, there was evidence of scar tissue in the portion of the tube joining the uterus. Other women had marked endometriosis which presumably had developed (or got worse) since a previous laparoscopy. Surgery produced several successful pregnancies, even in cases when IVF had already failed. Conclusion: about 15 per cent of unexplained infertility is due to tubal damage, or to severe endometriosis which was difficult to identify at an earlier laparoscopy.

● *Cervical problems.* Many couples had never undergone a post-coital test; alternatively, a negative post-coital test had been ignored or not followed up. Some of these women undoubtedly had a problem with their cervical mucus. Repeated tests were negative; in some cases, treatment resulted in the test becoming positive, although pregnancy rates remained rather discouragingly low. Conclusion: some unexplained infertility may be associated with a cervical mucus problem, though the precise importance of this is unclear.

● *Several minor factors together.* Some unexplained infertility is clearly the result of a number of subtle factors occurring together in the same couple. For example, where a man with 'marginal semen' marries a woman who ovulates slightly irregularly, they may be infertile. Marriage to different partners might have had an entirely different outcome.

● *Age.* We find far more 'unexplained' infertility in older couples. Presumably, these normal people have just reached the end of reproductive age a little earlier than normal, which is why we fail to find an obvious defect.

● *A genetic problem.* Several couples had an abnormal chromosome analysis. This affected either the man or woman and could not be treated directly. Furthermore, unexplained infertility may also result from a gene defect when the chromosomes look normal but carry an abnormal gene that cannot be detected. Conclusion: at least 2 per cent of unexplained infertility is due to a genetic defect.

What tests should be done if the infertility is unexplained?

I would strongly recommend that every reasonable effort be made to establish a diagnosis before complex treatments, such as IVF, are undertaken. Here is a list of the tests most commonly forgotten, or just undervalued. Some may well be worth carrying out for the first time or repeating it there is still doubt about the diagnosis.

FOR THE WOMAN

● *Good X-rays of the uterus* – hysterosalpingogram (HSG) – are really worth getting. The HSG gives information about the uterus and, to a lesser extent, the tubes which cannot be obtained by laparoscopy alone.

● *Hysteroscopy.* If there is any suspicion at all of an abnormal uterus, a telescope inspection of its interior is well worth while. Sometimes this reveals abnormalities that do not show well even on X-ray. When we suspect abnormalities of the uterus, especially its wall, we sometimes also take a tiny piece (biopsy) for microscopic examination.

● *Carefully timed post-coital tests* are often forgotten. They help to establish (1) whether there may be a problem, (2) whether there are antibodies to sperm in the cervical mucus and (3) whether there may be other problems in the cervix itself preventing manufacture of good mucus.

● *Repeated laparoscopy.* If a year or two has elapsed since the last inspection by laparoscopy, it may well be worth repeating it. If it is, it should be done by somebody with a keen interest in infertility and substantial experience. Photographs should be taken so that there is a permanent record of what exactly was seen.

● *Thorough hormone tests* done throughout the menstrual cycle. A study we have just completed shows that routine, single plasma progesterone tests – the most common test for ovulation – are only reliable 65 per cent of the time. Regular blood samples – particularly in the first half of the cycle (often neglected) and perhaps taken around the mid-cycle – may be needed to see if there are any subtle problems which might either affect ovulation, the quality of the eggs produced, or the uterine environment.

● *Ultrasound scans* of the ovaries. These should be done at the beginning of the menstrual cycle – occasionally requiring even four or five tests – to confirm that ovulation is really occurring and that there is no sign of polycystic ovaries.

FOR THE MAN

● *Repeated sperm counts*, over several months if necessary. Far too many men have just one count done. This is not sufficient for any serious investigation of infertility and certainly not enough if there is a somewhat obscure cause for it.

● *Sperm function tests*. Several different tests are coming into regular use. They include the sperm separation test (*see* p. 143), the zona attachment test, antibody tests, and the hamster test (*see* p. 145). Alternatively, some hospitals are now doing special examinations of sperm under an electron microscope. This powerful machine magnifies much more than a conventional microscope and may help to find a problem in some sperm.

FOR BOTH PARTNERS

● *Chromosome tests* on blood samples from both partners to see if there is any abnormality which might prevent a normal embryo being formed.

All these tests are well worth considering for those who have been told that their infertility cannot be explained. Certainly they should be discussed with the doctor, and if they can be done, I suggest making every possible attempt to establish the cause of the infertility as clearly as possible. In the next chapter, I discuss IVF and GIFT, treatments which are frequently offered to people with unexplained infertility. Both are stressful, emotionally demanding and physically invasive. Moreover, they are usually quite expensive. Before undertaking either of them it is definitely best first to try to establish the cause of the problem.

Thirty-nine-year-old Kathleen had been told by several doctors that her infertility was unexplained, and she was advised to have IVF and/or GIFT treatment. Because she was desperate (her marriage was not secure) and because she was quite well off, she underwent no fewer than seven attempts at IVF and three at GIFT in the next two years. All this treatment was done privately, and she tells me that in two years, she spent a total of £25,000. In all that time she never had an X-ray of her uterus to see if the cavity was normal. When I suggested this, the subsequent X-ray showed a large polyp. She came into hospital for the day and it was removed in an eight-minute procedure. She conceived two months later.

CHAPTER ELEVEN

Test-tube Babies and Similar Treatments

In vitro fertilisation

WHAT IS THE TEST-TUBE BABY TECHNIQUE?

Test-tube baby treatment is the popular name for in vitro fertilisation, usually shortened to IVF. Most people know what is meant by the term IVF, so I have used it exclusively. It is the process by which egg and sperm are mixed outside the body and then returned to the uterus after fertilisation. It involves the removal of an egg from the woman's ovary, the collection and purification of sperm from her partner, the mixing of sperm and egg in the laboratory and, if fertilisation occurs, the insertion of the developing fertilised egg – the embryo – into the uterus. The embryo, still quite invisible to the naked eye, is placed in its mother's uterus usually two days after fertilisation, while it still consists of only a few cells and long before any organs have formed.

WHAT ARE 'IN VITRO FERTILISATION', 'EXTRA–CORPOREAL FERTILISATION' AND 'EMBRYO TRANSFER'?

'In vitro fertilisation' really means fertilisation in glassware[28] (from *vitrum*, Latin for 'glass'). 'Extra-corporeal fertilisation' is

---

[28] In practice, IVF units hardly ever use glassware; plastic is much preferred because absolute cleanliness is essential. Washing glassware clean enough is

another term mostly used by those too obstinate to employ the more widely accepted terminology; it merely means fertilisation outside the body. 'Embryo transfer' is the process of placing the embryo into the mother's uterus.

Many people confuse 'artificial insemination' with IVF, but it is totally different. In artificial insemination, a doctor or nurse places sperm directly into a woman's vagina or uterus using a syringe or other artificial method, rather than conception occurring by natural intercourse; fertilisation occurs within the woman's Fallopian tube in the usual way. 'Assisted conception' is an increasingly widely used bit of jargon, employed to describe IVF and similar, related treatments.

THE STAGES OF IVF TREATMENT

1. TESTING A COUPLE'S SUITABILITY BEFORE TREATMENT

IVF is by no means suitable for every infertile couple. This vital aspect is often ignored. About half the women referred to IVF programmes could be more appropriately treated differently. Before treatment is started, several sperm counts, tests to discover the hormone levels and other procedures should be carried out to confirm whether there is a proper chance of success.[29] For example, the condition of the uterine cavity should be reviewed (perhaps by X-ray) if this has not been done recently; it is most important to make sure that the uterus is healthy enough to allow an embryo to implant and develop. The woman may sometimes be given drugs to make her ovulate so that her response to these drugs can be assessed well before an actual treatment cycle. This enables the medical team to tailor treatment to suit individual needs.

---

virtually impossible, so plastic dishes and equipment are used only once, fresh from the manufacturer and immediately thrown away. Nor for that matter are test-tubes used much; embryologists generally prefer to handle embryos in small dishes about 3 inches (7.5 cm) across.

[29] This list of tests is not exhaustive, and does not include the preliminary tests which should be done in all infertile couples before treatment of any sort.

2. STIMULATION OF OVULATION

The best chance of successful pregnancy is obtained when more than one embryo is placed in the uterus at the same time. This is because so many early human embryos, normally fertilised, are lost or do not develop into babies. Consequently, one way of overcoming this natural loss is to put back several embryos simultaneously during IVF. When two or three embryos are put back together, the risk of a multiple pregnancy such as twins is not that great though it is certainly high enough to be a cause of real concern.

In order to obtain more than one embryo, more than one egg is needed. This is why drugs such as clomiphene (Clomid) or HMG (Humegon or Pergonal) are given to make the ovaries work harder than normal. Occasionally, many eggs are obtained simultaneously with these drugs but it is very uncommon for all of them to fertilise and form into normal embryos.

One of these drugs will normally be given to the woman (in the form of either an injection or pills) a few days after her period, at the start of the treatment cycle. The dose and the length of time these drugs are given may be deliberately varied, depending on her individual response. Recently, many IVF centres have been using so-called 'programmed cycles'. This ensures that the doctors have a greater degree of control over the ovaries, just temporarily, which may allow more precise timing of when eggs should be collected. The evidence suggests that this approach can improve the results of IVF. Many clinics are also giving the drug buserelin (Suprefact) in addition to HMG. As we have seen (*see* p. 175) buserelin prevents the pituitary gland from sending messages to the ovaries, and this means that the ovaries respond more effectively to the HMG treatment given subsequently. This seems to result in more eggs being produced simultaneously, with a higher pregnancy rate in certain cases. Other clinics use progestogens (synthetic forms of progesterone), which are cheaper and may give results which are nearly as good. Buserelin can be given in various ways: some clinics give it just for a few days (the so-called 'short protocol') before starting HMG, and some give it for about two weeks (so-called 'long protocol') before starting ovarian stimulation with Humegon or Pergonal. The long protocol is generally better, but as it uses more drugs it is more expensive.

3. ASSESSING THE DEVELOPMENT OF THE EGGS

Egg collection is generally timed to within a few hours of when the woman is expected to ovulate. If eggs are not collected very close to this time, they may not fertilise properly. This is the main reason why so many tests are often done to confirm the status of the woman's hormones and, thus, development of her eggs.

There are basically three ways by which the chance of collecting mature eggs can be improved. None is wholly accurate, and a good deal of experience is needed to pinpoint the moment before ovulation.

● *Hormone tests.* As the follicle swells, the hormones oestrogen and progesterone are produced in increasing amounts. Regular blood tests can detect this increase. Also, provided the woman is not taking buserelin, the pituitary gland in the brain produces luteinising hormone (LH), which gives a message to the ovary to start the ovulation process. This hormone can also be detected in the blood. Unfortunately, not all clinics perform regular hormone tests during stimulation. This is a pity, because regular hormone tests are extremely helpful in getting the best results and because analysis of the hormone results after a failed treatment cycle can give crucial information about how to improve the treatment if another cycle of IVF is contemplated.

● *Ultrasound.* The swelling follicle can be directly measured using ultrasound (*see* p. 149). This is usually done daily. We know from experience that, when the follicle is about 20 millimetres across, ovulation is imminent. Most clinics now use vaginal ultrasound – the ultrasound probe, instead of being placed on the abdomen, is inserted gently into the vagina. Most of our patients greatly prefer this: they can take an intelligent interest in what their doctor is seeing on the screen, without bursting to go to the toilet. Moreover, ultrasound measurement using a vaginal probe is more accurate.

● *Injection of HCG* shortly before ovulation would normally occur. This gives a message to the ovary to start the process by which the follicle ruptures and ovulation itself happens. Normally ovulation will occur about thirty-seven hours after the injection and egg collection must be done before this time has elapsed. The injection of HCG also initiates the chemical processes in the egg which ripens it before a woman ovulates. It is usually only used if the pituitary gland has not yet started to produce LH or if the woman is taking buserelin.

The timing of the HCG injection and subsequent egg collection is fairly critical. If egg collection is left too late, the eggs may be lost. If collection is done too soon, the eggs will not have had time to mature properly and therefore may not fertilise normally. This is one of the reasons why repeated hormone tests during IVF are important – to time the proper moment for the HCG and for the subsequent egg collection.

NATURAL CYCLES

A few centres often do not give any major stimulus to the ovaries during IVF at all, beyond a single injection of HCG to trigger ovulation. This must still be accurately timed. Without stimulation usually only one egg can be collected. This makes natural cycle treatment cheaper because injections of ovulatory drugs are expensive. Moreover, transferring only one embryo avoids the risk of twins. However, natural cycle IVF is not generally as successful, because there are fewer embryos produced and usually only one for transfer.

4. EGG COLLECTION

Eggs may occasionally be collected by laparoscopy, in which case a general anaesthetic is given. More usually, the eggs are collected using ultrasound, normally vaginal ultrasound. In this method, a picture of the ovaries is obtained by means of a thin ultrasound probe placed in the vagina. A needle is placed through the top of the vagina and guided into the ovary; eggs are then sucked from the follicles into a small test-tube which is immediately handed to the embryologist to examine.[30] This is a very convenient technique, frequently involving only a light anaesthetic or merely a little local anaesthetic with sedation. In good clinics, this method is seldom accompanied by any real pain. We find that most of our own patients much prefer the vaginal approach, under local anaesthetic. If local anaesthesia is used, the woman has to be in hospital for only a few hours.

In spite of the great care that is taken, it is not always possible to get all the eggs (or sometimes even a single egg). However, in good centres, 97 per cent of attempts at egg collection yield at least one egg, unless there is very severe disease of the ovaries, so the risk of total failure at this stage is small.

5. EGG CULTURE, SPERM PREPARATION AND FERTILISATION

Once the eggs have been collected, they can be easily damaged. They are carefully identified under a microscope in the operating theatre suite and then immediately placed in specially prepared fluid. This fluid – the culture medium – contains very precisely measured amounts of the chemicals needed for the eggs' survival as well as some of the woman's own serum previously obtained from a routine sample of her blood.

The eggs in their culture medium are then put into an incubator. This is simply a kind of oven, which will keep the eggs at exactly the right temperature under rigidly controlled

[30] In the early days of IVF when the achievement of collecting each egg was a matter of wonderment and congratulation, laparoscopic egg collection under general anaesthesia was complicated and took a long time. Struggling for over seventy minutes to collect just one egg at a particularly awkward procedure, I managed eventually to puncture a second follicle, obtaining another egg. Triumphantly handing the open test-tube to the embryologist, we were both suddenly conscious of how long the patient had been unconscious. 'What's the time, Steve?' I said to the embryologist, now very much one of Europe's leading reproductive scientists. 'About two hours,' said Steve, automatically inverting his wrist to look at his watch. We both stood appalled as the precious contents of the tube splashed on to the floor. Within seconds, everybody got on their hands and knees, looking for the totally invisible egg. Remarkably, Mrs B got pregnant with the one egg.

conditions which resemble those within the body as closely as possible.

Usually shortly before the eggs are collected, the man will be asked to produce semen by masturbation. A bedroom is available in most clinics for this purpose. Men often find this part of IVF very worrying – it is quite common to find that a man simply cannot ejaculate under this kind of emotional pressure. If this is likely to be a problem, most good units will make arrangements to freeze and store semen samples before treatment, ready for use. Unfortunately, semen that has been frozen and then thawed is not usually as fertile as freshly produced semen.

Once the semen has been produced, the sperm are washed and diluted in the laboratory, and the number of sperm are counted under a microscope. Several hours after egg collection, they will be mixed with the culture medium containing the eggs and these will then be replaced in the incubator. Unfortunately, it is not uncommon to find a last-minute problem with the sperm: they may be too few in number or too weak in other ways. At present, most IVF programmes need several thousand normal sperm to guarantee fertilisation of even a single egg.

6. EMBRYO CULTURE

In a good IVF unit, the cultured eggs will be inspected under a microscope about eighteen hours after they have been mixed with the sperm, and again after about 24–30 hours. The reason for the inspection at eighteen hours is that this may be the only time that definite signs of fertilisation may be observed. The egg may actually divide into several cells later on, without ever having been fertilised. This is called *parthenogenetic cleavage* (*see* p. 29) and in clinics that are not very effective, there is a risk that unfertilised, parthenogenetically cleaved eggs may be transferred to the uterus. These, of course, give no chance of normal pregnancy.

The embryo will usually have divided into about 2–4 cells after forty-eight hours, although occasionally growth may be more advanced than this. Before an embryo is transferred to the uterus, the scientists check to make sure it appears normal. If there is doubt about this, they may suggest waiting for a further twenty-four hours before a decision is taken about its transfer. In good units, transfer sixty hours after fertilisation, rather than forty-eight hours, does not affect success. If an embryo seems seriously abnormal, it is discarded, rather than run the slightest risk of a damaged pregnancy. Needless to say, the great majority of units allow women to go home after egg collection, so that the decision to recall them for an embryo transfer can be made after observing how the embryos have developed.

7. EMBRYO TRANSFER

When an embryo is ready to be put back into the womb, it is loaded into fine plastic tubing, together with a minute drop of culture fluid. After the woman is vaginally examined briefly, the tubing is inserted through her cervix. The fluid containing the embryo (or embryos, if there are more than one) is now squirted extremely gently into the uterus. This is normally very easy indeed and, as it is not only painless but usually not even felt, it hardly ever requires an anaesthetic. Nearly all clinics usually put the embryos into the uterus with the woman lying on her back. Once the embryo transfer has been done, most clinics ask the woman to remain lying down for thirty minutes or even possibly longer. It is thought that this may help the embryo to 'stay put', but there is no good evidence for this.

Injections (or suppositories) of progesterone, or occasionally injections of HCG, are frequently given to the woman after embryo transfer. This is thought by some to help a pregnancy to implant, but there is much doubt whether it really helps.

At this stage, once an embryo has been transferred, nearly all women are naturally nervous about what they can or cannot do. After embryo transfer, many are so anxious that they might lose the early embryos that they lie rigid in bed for hours at a time.[31] This is quite unnecessary – all that is suggested is lying

[31] One other thing that units do which often causes patients great anxiety is, just before transfer, to grade the embryos visually under the microscope, and

horizontal for thirty minutes or so. In any case, embryos do not immediately implant after transfer; this takes place several days later, and there is no evidence that this is influenced by routine activities. If implantation was influenced by a woman moving around, then clearly nobody would ever get pregnant, particularly if energetic sexual activity took place. People should definitely not regard themselves as invalids, but because of these understandable worries it seems quite reasonable to take things easy for a few days, perhaps staying off work for two or three days, and avoiding sex for two weeks. There is categorically no need to stay in bed. However, there is no evidence that even these simple precautions make much difference. On the other hand, overseas travel is best avoided for two weeks, if possible, in order to keep in close contact with the clinic that did the IVF treatment.

8. PREGNANCY TESTING

Although everything up to this stage may have gone quite easily and embryos were put into the uterus without difficulty, the chances are high that the woman will not get pregnant. Many embryos are lost before the menstrual period is due, and this can be extremely disappointing. The reasons for these failures are not clear but it is likely that many embryos which look normal under an ordinary laboratory microscope are poorly developed and just not capable of producing a pregnancy. This is not surprising as many human embryos produced naturally during normal 'fertile' cycles simply are incapable of subsequent development. Much research is being done about this, as we shall see in the last chapter.

Some clinics do not test for pregnancy at all; others suggest that the woman sends them a urine sample if she wishes. At Hammersmith we normally take some blood from most patients

---

then tell women that they have got 'good' embryos or 'not so good' embryos. There is no way that visual inspection will give any reasonable information about embryo quality, unless the embryos are so bad that they should not be returned to the uterus at all.

on the twelfth and fourteenth day after embryo transfer – the earliest that a very small pregnancy can be detected.

ARE THERE RISKS TO IVF? WILL THE BABY BE NORMAL?

At the time of writing, about 20,000 babies have been born around the world following IVF, and they show that there is no special risk of abnormality. One in every fifty babies born after natural conception has an abnormality of some sort. This risk is not increased after IVF; indeed, there is some evidence that certain types of abnormality (such as chromosome problems, for example Down's syndrome) are actually less common after IVF. There have been suggestions that IVF babies tend to have more problems at birth and that stillbirths are very slightly more common. This apparent trend is not due to the IVF but probably because many infertile women (who end up with successful treatment) are in the 'high-risk' group. Also, IVF frequently results in multiple pregnancy (e.g., twins) which carries a higher risk of problems with babies, such as premature delivery.

WHAT IS THE RISK OF TWINS OR TRIPLETS?

IVF is less successful unless more than one embryo is transferred simultaneously, but the more embryos that are transferred at once, the greater the chance of twins, triplets or even more. This is why the number of transferred embryos should be limited. Many infertile women, after years of forlorn treatment, are only too ready to accept such risks. In most clinics the chance of a twin pregnancy is about 25 per cent. Whilst twins are not too difficult to deal with, triplets are undoubtedly best avoided, and quadruplets are really a disaster. Apart from the risks of a premature delivery, bringing up so many babies at once places a great burden on a family. The best IVF units always limit the number of embryos transferred simultaneously, even if this means slightly reduced success. Good units (because of their control procedures and the quality of the embryos they produce) need to transfer fewer embryos to get good success rates.

IS THERE ANY PHYSICAL RISK TO THE WOMAN?

Very occasionally the drugs given to stimulate the ovaries may cause too many follicles to develop. This may result in the ovaries becoming temporarily swollen and cystic – the so-called hyperstimulation syndrome – a condition which often requires hospital admission but usually settles down after a few days' bedrest. The main risk is associated with egg collection, which, however trivial, is still a surgical procedure. Most people are pretty scared of anaesthesia, but the fact that the better IVF units are in proper hospitals or clinics should give ample reassurance. Ultrasonic egg collection is no more risky than a laparoscopy.

DO THE DRUGS CAUSE CANCER?

Some irresponsible people, regrettably some doctors, have seriously frightened patients by suggesting that the drugs given to stimulate ovulation may cause cancer of the ovary or breast. Most of the people who say this disapprove of IVF for quite different reasons and may try to give their criticisms more weight by making these suggestions. Superovulatory drugs such as Clomid and HMG have been in regular use in large amounts for thirty-five years, before IVF treatment was even a possibility. During that time no studies at all have clearly shown any relationship whatsoever between cancer and the use of these drugs. Both Clomid and HMG have not been shown to have any serious long-term side-effects and the various national committees which control their use are fully satisfied that they are safe.

WILL WE BE ABLE TO STAND THE EMOTIONAL STRAIN?

Some people find in vitro fertilisation very demanding emotionally. Both women and men always find it more stressful than they expect. Having to go to the hospital regularly, the inevitable waiting around, travelling and staying away from home, the monitoring of follicle growth all result in tension and worry. The build-up to egg collection, with the possible admission to hospital and the waiting time until embryo transfer (assuming this is possible) require considerable fortitude. In addition, it is often not easy for the man to produce his semen at the moment of egg collection. Once the embryo has been put back in the uterus the situation can be even more fraught because the chances are that the woman's period will come on within the next two weeks. Not infrequently, this occurs after a delay of a few days or so and, of course, this can be quite devastating.

These real problems are a fact of treatment, and it is most important that couples should only enter treatment if they feel strong enough to bear those kinds of shocks and the waiting that it involves. It is also important that couples should support one another; many find an added strength in their relationship at times like this.

CAN THE TREATMENT BE REPEATED?

This largely depends on the response to the previous IVF treatment attempt. It occasionally becomes clear that no amount of hormone therapy or treatment for deficiencies in the sperm (both relatively common examples) will make IVF successful. Under these or similar circumstances, IVF should probably not be repeated. Sometimes such decisions can be re-evaluated months or even years later, if there have been any hopeful scientific or medical developments. Most clinics will repeat the treatment for suitable patients, although some set a limit of about three or four attempts. In the private sector, it generally depends on how one feels and whether couples feel confident that they can stand the upheaval – and if they have the money.

'TRANSPORT IVF'

There are many variations of how IVF treatment may be done. One of the problems about IVF is that it is not cheap. It also involves women in attending a hospital which may be a considerable distance from their home, at very frequent intervals. A few centres have established transport IVF to overcome these problems. This involves collaboration between a local hospital and a central IVF unit.

The woman attends her local hospital for the earlier stages of treatment which involve stimulation of ovulation and egg collection. She has regular ultrasound in the usual way, and should have hormone tests to time the egg collection. Following egg collection at her local hospital, the woman rests until she is ready to return home. Once the eggs have been collected they are placed in a small portable twelve-volt incubator. This incubator is kept at the right temperature electrically by plugging its power supply into the cigar lighter of a car. Fortunately, a Rolls Royce is not necessary to own a cigar lighter these days. The husband then drives to the central IVF unit where the eggs are removed from the car incubator. Here he produces a semen sample and the eggs are fertilised. Two days later the woman can come at leisure to the central IVF unit where an embryo transfer is done. This treatment has the advantage of reducing the number of long journeys that a woman normally makes to a central IVF unit, and because all laboratory facilities are centralised, it reduces the cost of treatment. We are starting this treatment at Hammersmith and are collaborating with other hospitals in our region; it is too early to say whether results are comparable with fully centralised IVF. However in Liverpool, where this treatment has been going on for some time, doctors and patients there are very pleased with the results.

This idea was pioneered in France a few years ago by Professor Bernard Hedon in Montpellier, who provides a central IVF laboratory for five outlying hospitals, two of which are more than 94 miles (150 km) distant. In Montpellier they have had excellent results. Professor Hedon told me that the husbands did not mind the long drive into Montpellier and that they got down the motorway within an hour, in time to hand in the eggs. When I suggested that they must be going incredibly fast and breaking the speed limit, he replied, with a pout and an expressive French shrug, 'Ah, but they look forward to producing the sperm when they reach the end of the journey.' So far there has been no problem with the traffic police in the south of France.

WHEN SHOULD IVF BE CONSIDERED?

The main situations when IVF may be worth considering are:

● When the tubes are badly damaged and tubal surgery has less chance of success than IVF, or in most cases where tubal surgery has already been unsuccessful. IVF should be considered because it bypasses the tubes.

● When the man's sperm count is on the low side or abnormal, yet potentially capable of fertilising an egg. Here IVF may be useful because fertilisation can possibly be manipulated and observed by the scientific team. This does not necessarily require sperm injection, or zona drilling, but simply very careful preparation of the sperm in suitable laboratory solutions.

● For certain women who have problems with the cervix, perhaps 'hostile' mucus, IVF bypasses the cervix and its mucus.

● For women who are not ovulating spontaneously, but who produce eggs on fertility drugs without conceiving. In this situation, the ability to force the ovary to produce many eggs and then select the best ones for fertilisation and transfer means that IVF may be a suitable option.

● For some women with endometriosis or with very carefully investigated infertility which remains unexplained. We think that endometriosis is an excellent indication for IVF and have had particular success.

● For couples who have several factors together which are causing infertility; commonly a combination of poor male fertility and tubal disease are the most usual indications.

● Most recently, for certain couples who are at high risk of having genetically abnormal babies.

WHO IS UNSUITABLE FOR IN VITRO FERTILISATION?

Unfortunately, there are many couples who have one of the problems listed above for whom even IVF is of no help. These include women who:

● have had the uterus removed (*hysterectomy*);
● have severe scarring or abnormalities of the uterus (such as very bad adenomyosis), making pregnancy impossible;
● have had tuberculosis (or another serious infection) of the uterus which has left very bad scar tissue;
● have very scarred or extensive cystic ovaries. It may be impossible to collect a healthy egg, even though ovulation is occurring;
● have very severe bowel adhesions around the ovaries which could make even ultrasonic egg collection very dangerous;
● are much over about forty-three years old, when IVF is notoriously unsuccessful. However there are signs that IVF may become increasingly successful in older women.

In addition, IVF is nearly always impossible if the man's sperm count is lower than 100,000.

IVF AND MALE INFERTILITY

MICRODROPLET CULTURE

There are a number of techniques that have been attempted to overcome a low sperm count. Several units have tried placing the eggs in very small volumes of fluid with the sperm. This technique may help fertilisation rates by concentrating all the available sperm closely around the egg. When the man's vas deferens is damaged or blocked, a very few units have had very limited success by fertilising eggs in droplets of fluid containing sperm taken by needle aspiration from the man's epididymis. At present, such a sophisticated approach is very experimental.

DISSOLVING OR DRILLING THE ZONA

There has been great interest recently in attempts to improve fertilisation rates by manipulating egg and sperm together during IVF treatment. Two main approaches have been employed by research workers around the world. The first has been to dissolve the outer shell of the human egg – the zona – using enzymes or acid solutions. This has the theoretical advantage that sperm which are not very motile might be capable of penetrating the softer, 'business' parts of the egg and forming an embryro. Embryos have resulted from this method, but there is still a question mark over their normality. Total removal of the zona may leave the egg so unprotected that it becomes infected by any viruses which may be around; this would be highly undesirable as it may possibly lead to an abnormal baby. Another problem is that we do not know whether a reasonably intact zona is required for normal embryonic development.

Because total removal of the zona seems essentially unsafe, other workers have tried drilling microscopic holes in the zona. It is thought that sperm might get through these holes rather more easily than through zonas that are intact. Researchers have been successful in getting such eggs to fertilise. However, fertilisation has been pretty erratic, and to date only a few human embryos have resulted in successful pregnancies.

SPERM MANIPULATION AND INJECTION INTO THE EGG

An alternative approach has been the deliberate injection of sperm into the egg, using a sophisticated microscope and micromanipulators. The egg is quite invisible, so such microsurgery requires quite complex equipment. The egg is immobilised by sucking it on to an extremely fine pipette, and a minute stab wound is made with a remarkably fine glass tube. A single sperm is chosen and then injected into the egg. In Australia several animal pregnancies have been reported with this technique. In Britain, this promising technique has been largely pioneered by Dr Simon Fishel, of Nurture, at Nottingham University. He is a world authority on sperm injection and has

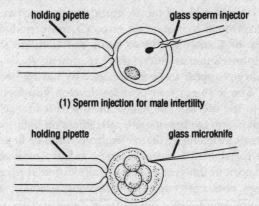

(1) Sperm injection for male infertility

(2) Embryo biopsy for genetic diagnosis

Micromanipulation. These experimental techniques may be for: (1) Sperm injection. The egg is held by a glass-holding pipette using gentle suction; sperm injection is done with a very fine glass tube; or (2) a six- or eight-cell embryo has one cell removed through a minute hole made by a glass microknife. This cell will then be subjected to chemical analysis.

had the most success with this treatment. At the time of writing, I understand that about thirty babies have been born after sperm injection, or SUZI (subzonal injection) as Dr Fishel calls it. However, there is still quite a long way to go before this can become a widely used clinical treatment and it is somewhat experimental. One of the problems is that we have no idea how to select a healthy sperm for injection; this technique could possibly force unhealthy sperm into an egg with unforeseen results.

EMBRYO FREEZING

Embryos can be stored for long periods of time at very low temperatures. Much of this technology was developed by Professor David Whittingham and Professor Chris Polge, well-known English scientists working in Cambridge and at the Medical Research Council in the 1970s. David Whittingham has stored a large number of mouse embryos for over twenty years in liquid nitrogen (temperature −196°C) and periodically takes a number of them out, thaws them and transfers them to a suitable mouse's uterus. Successive experiments show that these mice embryos appear to be undamaged by having been in cold storage. About 80 per cent of them develop into foetuses after transfer to the uterus. The length of time that mouse embryos have been in storage has no particular effect on their viability. It seems, in all probability, that an embryo could be kept in liquid nitrogen for several hundred years; a baby conceived in 1993 could be born in the year 2293 to totally different parents. This technology does raise curious ethical considerations, and some bizarre ones; one's aunt could also be one's niece – work that out!

Freezing technology, or *cryopreservation*, has now been applied to other animal species and is increasingly widely used for some species of cattle, cows, horses and sheep, for example. It is very useful for various forms of animal husbandry and, amongst other applications, means that embryos from a particular stock of animals can conveniently be transported around the world to start new herds. There may be other important uses for this technology in future, such as preservation of endangered species. However, one problem with this technology is that embryos of different species require different methods of freezing for success. Indeed, scientists have been unable successfully to freeze and store embryos of a number of different species. This does have important implications when embryo freezing is applied in humans.

HOW IS EMBRYO FREEZING DONE?

For embryos to be kept for longer periods than relatively few hours, they need to be kept at very low temperatures, much lower than a normal refrigerator. An analogy is the domestic refrigerator; food kept more than a few days or a week will start to go off, and even foodstuffs in a deep freeze, at, say, −20°C, go off with time. Very low temperatures thus are needed for live human or animal cells, and in this respect liquid nitrogen is ideal. At −196°C there is no demonstrable deterioration. However, uncontrolled cooling, even at room temperatures, of any embryo may cause very severe damage to it. This damage may include damage to the chromosomes so that the embryo is incapable of subsequent development. Because all cells contain water, cooling below the freezing point of water produces ice-crystal formation inside the embryo. This may not matter too much during the freezing process, but certainly is of critical importance during thawing. This is because as ice melts, it expands. This expansion causes severe damage to the embryo, breaking it up. This is similar to damage to frozen pipes in winter, during a thaw.

In order to prevent cooling injury, various cryoprotectants chemicals have been employed before the freezing process. These tend to prevent ice recrystallisation when embryos are subsequently thawed after preservation. The most well-known is glycerol, similar in some respects to the antifreeze used in a car radiator. Other compounds which have been used successfully include dimethylsulphoxide and propanediol.

WHAT ARE THE ADVANTAGES OF EMBRYO FREEZING?

IVF frequently involves the production of more embryos than can be safely transferred to the uterus simultaneously. Preservation of any spare embryos means that a woman can have these thawed later and transferred if she does not first get pregnant with her fresh embryos. Frozen embryos can also be used for donation to other infertile couples if the donor gets pregnant and no longer wants her embryos for her own treatment. Embryo freezing may also be used to preserve the embryos of married women who may be undergoing treatments for malignant diseases, such as cancer or leukaemia. Freezing is valuable because these treatments may cause sterility, often preventing women from producing eggs subsequently.

WHAT ARE THE DISADVANTAGES OF EMBRYO FREEZING?

Although many clinics seem wildly enthusiastic about freezing, there are several reasons why I firmly believe that human embryo freezing should be treated with real caution.

1. When carefully analysed, the results of frozen-thawed embryo transfer are not particularly good. The technology may fail at several stages. First, not all human embryos will freeze successfully, as the freezing process often results in their total destruction. Quite frequently, apparently normal embryos will not survive thawing, either. At the last global count, published at a recent world congress on in vitro fertilisation, only about 2.5 per cent of frozen embryos subsequently gave rise to fully viable pregnancies. Admittedly some IVF clinics have done better than this, but there is no doubt that thawed embryos are not as 'good' as fresh ones.

2. Stored spare embryos, taken from the IVF cycle, which did not produce a successful pregnancy after fresh embryo transfer, are even less likely to result in pregnancy. The success of IVF depends primarily on the quality of the embryos transferred, and hence on the quality of the eggs which preceded the embryos. In a given cycle, any spare 'sibling' eggs and embryos will have been matured in the same hormonal environment. A failed treatment cycle implies that the spare embryos that are preserved are likely to be of even less good quality than those which were transferred.

3. Embryo freezing is labour-intensive, and therefore costly to carry out. It is not unusual for clinics to charge up to £500 to freeze embryos, perhaps more to store them for long periods and occasionally even more to transfer them. With a relatively low success rate, it is certainly more cost-effective (though perhaps not so convenient) to go through a complete new cycle from scratch.

4. Embryo freezing may possibly carry genuine risks to the foetus. Although many animals have been born without any mishap, and quite a few humans, the use of cryoprotectants which are needed causes misgivings. I certainly would not want to take any of these chemicals by mouth and, of course, all

doctors are worried about exposing any woman to drugs during early pregnancy for fear of causing malformation. I must emphasize that no abnormalities in the foetus or baby have ever been attributed to freezing. Nevertheless, it was nearly forty years before we realised that exposure to ionising radiation during early pregnancy could result in leukaemia in subsequent childhood. Experience with human embryo freezing is relatively short, and I therefore feel that this technology should still be regarded as somewhat experimental.

WHEN SHOULD EMBRYO FREEZING BE CONTEMPLATED?

In our unit, at the time of writing, we are reluctant to offer routine embryo freezing. We still feel that caution is appropriate, only generally offering it when there is no clear alternative.

1. Embryo freezing seems reasonable when a woman needs cancer treatment which may make her infertile. Nowadays, most young women survive radiation for leukaemia or cancer of the lymph glands, or various forms of chemotherapy. Often the sterility caused by this treatment results in more distress than the thought that the cancer may not be cured. Under such circumstances, it seems reasonable to offer cryopreservation.

2. Very occasionally, a woman may become ill during the IVF. Embryo transfer and pregnancy may make her condition worse. Under such circumstances, it seems reasonable to preserve the embryos until she has fully recovered, allowing an embryo transfer some months later.

3. Women over forty years old undergoing IVF are in an especially difficult situation. Often, they simply cannot afford to wait for another IVF attempt if the first one fails. Under these circumstances, I think the risks of embryo freezing are possibly outweighed by the advantages, because any spare stored frozen embryos could be thawed and transferred at monthly intervals afterwards.

4. For people receiving donor embryo treatment. Before an embryo is transferred into the uterus a period of quarantine is

indicated to ensure that the donor does not have serious disease such as AIDS.

EGG FREEZING

Egg freezing offers great hope for the future. It would be a tremendous advance if we could store eggs safely. This would be useful for women who might be made sterile by various medical treatments but who are unmarried without a regular partner. When they do eventually marry they obviously would like to have their own genetic offspring. Egg freezing would also be of enormous benefit for treating women with donated eggs (see Chapter 12), allowing those young women with a premature menopause more access to effective treatment.

Various attempts to freeze both human and animal eggs have been made. There seems no doubt that eventually the problems with egg freezing will be solved but, presently, egg freezing is more difficult and dangerous than embryo freezing. Exposure to cold can induce severe genetic damage to mammalian eggs which may incur chromosome damage during the freezing process. A few normal mice have been born after egg freezing, but the success rates are much lower than with embryo cryopreservation. Some highly abnormal mice have also been born after egg freezing. To date, only two human births have followed egg freezing. These babies were normal, but there have been some miscarriages possibly as a result of genetic abnormality. Scientists are universally agreed that egg freezing must still be regarded as experimental until more research work has been done on the embryos which are produced after various egg freezing attempts.

WHAT FACTORS ARE ASSOCIATED WITH IVF SUCCESS?

What causes success in some cases and failure in others is not known. However, certain factors are associated with a normal pregnancy after IVF. These include:

● The establishment of a really good IVF laboratory which is expertly run with proper quality control.[32]

● Transfer of more than one embryo simultaneously.

● The age of the woman. Those over thirty–eight do less well. If a woman does get pregnant at forty by IVF, the chance of a miscarriage is higher than normal.

● Careful hormonal measurements. Careful control of hormone levels gives a better chance and they are particularly important in timing the HCG injection. Unfortunately many IVF centres do rather limited hormone testing, largely to save money. This may mean that the success rate may be lower. Moreover, if the eggs fail to fertilise and tests have not been done, it may not be possible to say whether they failed to fertilise because the hormones were just not adequate in that cycle of treatment, or whether there was some other problem – for example, with the sperm. This can be a big problem if further treatment is subsequently considered.

● The ability to collect eggs around the clock, seven days a week. Although this puts a huge strain on the staff and requires special efforts, the ability to collect eggs night or day, holidays included, has advantages for the woman.

WHAT ARE THE REASONS FOR FAILURE?

Even when patients are selected carefully, there are many pitfalls. Failure can occur at any stage. Unfortunately, the further that treatment has proceeded, the harder it is to accept

---

[32] Quality control is crucial because human embryos develop poorly in the wrong environment. In 1983, we realised that embryos are exquisitely sensitive to volatile oils. Painters decorating a hospital corridor released compounds from the emulsion paint they were using, completely inhibiting embryo growth in a locked laboratory well over 100 metres away. We have also found that some commercially available catheters used for embryo transfer killed every single embryo with which they came into contact. Since that time batches of all equipment which might meet an embryo are routinely cultured with animal embryos before releasing them for human use. Nor do we allow our laboratory personnel to wear perfume or aftershave. Smoking near the unit is also strictly forbidden.

failure, particularly if everything had seemed to be going well. The reasons for failure include:

● The ovaries may not produce a suitable follicle or follicles in the cycle during treatment. Alternatively, one of the ovaries may become enlarged temporarily with a cyst. If either of these things happen, treatment may have to be abandoned. In most cases, it will be possible to restart treatment after a period of resting the ovaries. Between 8 and 20 per cent of treatment cycles are abandoned, depending on the programme, so this is quite common. Very often treatment later in another month will result in an improved response.

● Eggs cannot be collected from the follicles at the time of laparoscopy or ultrasound. This accounts for less than 5 per cent of failures.

● The eggs fail to fertilise. This occurs in about 10 per cent of patients. The sperm may just not be healthy enough on the day of egg collection; this can happen even when many previous sperm counts haven't revealed a problem. Unfortunately, male infertility is almost certainly the most common reason for IVF to fail totally.

● The embryo or embryos fail to develop normally and have to be discarded. Perhaps 40 per cent of embryos fall into this category.

● An embryo or embryos are transferred to the uterus, but they don't implant. This is the most common reason for failure, occurring 70 per cent of the time. Just why apparently entirely healthy-looking embryos don't implant is still something of a mystery.

● The embryo implants and pregnancy commences, but a miscarriage occurs within a few weeks. Alternatively, in 6 per cent of cases, the pregnancy lodges in the tube (an ectopic pregnancy) from where it needs to be removed surgically. The incidence of miscarriage varies greatly from clinic to clinic – usually somewhere between 15 and 30 per cent.

IF IVF IS SO SUCCESSFUL, WHY BOTHER WITH OTHER TREATMENTS?

One of the most unsatisfactory aspects of IVF, and indeed all the newer reproductive techniques, is the way in which they have been promoted. In the fourteen or so years since Louise Brown, the world's first IVF baby, was conceived, most ordinary people, many journalists and not a few doctors have come to believe that IVF has been the greatest step forward in infertility treatment, virtually replacing all others. This impression is utterly wrong and the reality is different. IVF is still the most demanding, the most emotionally fraught, the most expensive, and one of the least successful of infertility treatments. More importantly, it is also one of the least available.

What is the evidence for these very provocative statements? Whichever way the success of IVF is examined, one has to say that results in many units are still very disappointing. Each year, the Licensing Authority for in vitro fertilisation and embryology has collected and collated the results from all the IVF clinics across Britain. This controlling body is now called the Human Fertilisation and Embryology Authority (HFEA, *see* pp. 340–1), and regulates by Act of Parliament. Although Britain is one of the most successful countries doing IVF, the reports of the HFEA clearly show how limited is this success. At the time of writing, the most recent annual report on British results was published in July 1992. This report states that in 1990 (the most recent year for which statistics are available):

● only 12.5 per cent of all IVF treatments produced a live baby;

● IVF units treating fewer than 400 women were even less successful;

● only 9,964 women in Britain were treated by IVF;

● 8 British IVF centres were responsible for the majority of pregnancies; the remaining 56 centres were usually less successful;

● only 1,443 live births occurred after IVF in the year 1990–91.

CLINIC SIZE*	PATIENTS	IVF CYCLES	PREGNANCIES	BIRTHS
Large (8)	5,218	6,165	1,198 (19.4%)	876 (14.2%)
Medium (21)	3,184	4,365	672 (15.4%)	484 (11.1%)
Small (35)	932	1,053	134 (12.7%)	83 (7.9%)
TOTAL:	9,964	11,583	2,004 (17.3)	1,443 (12.5%)

*Clinic size: This refers to the number of IVF treatments done annually. There were 8 large clinics performing over 400 cycles annually, 21 medium-size clinics performing 100–400 cycles, and 35 small clinics doing fewer than 100 cycles annually. Although large centres were on the whole more successful, there was considerable variability even amongst these; the least successful of the large IVF clinics only had 2.7 per cent success per cycle, with only 2.1 per cent live births. Some of the smallest clinics had had no pregnancies at all.

These statistics are gruesome. For one thing, clearly IVF is not nearly as successful as many people imagine. Second, one's chances of successful treatment depend very considerably on which clinic one chooses; although large clinics gave superior results on the whole, some large clinics did very badly and some smaller clinics did better than average: consequently, going to a large clinic is not a guarantee of getting the best treatment. Third, only a tiny proportion (less than 10,000) of Britain's infertile population received IVF treatment in 1990–91.

Although nowadays it is extremely difficult to adopt a baby in Britain, in 1990–91 almost as many couples successfully adopted a baby as those who had a baby born by IVF. Perhaps this, as much as any other statistic, focuses attention on just how unsuccessful IVF really is.

In view of all this, you may appreciate why I believe that the wide press coverage given to IVF is so unfortunate. Promotion of it has taken attention away from other treatments which are still usually far more helpful. A fraction of the investment given over to IVF would, if spent in other areas of infertility, undoubtedly produce more babies. Many academic units of obstetrics and gynaecology argue that they pursue IVF because of its value in research. Actually, remarkably little really innovative or valuable research emanates from the majority of IVF units, academic or private.

In my opinion, IVF baby treatment is still, with some notable exceptions, the last resort, useful only when a diagnosis indicating it has been firmly established or when all else has failed. Even then, it is quite definitely not suitable for all cases when other treatments have failed. At Hammersmith Hospital where we treat about 1,500 cycles each year, we only consider offering this treatment if there is some chance of success, however small. We feel very strongly that other treatments, being generally more successful, must usually be tried first, and that IVF should be reserved for when there is no realistic alternative and after every attempt has been made to establish a cause for the infertility.

All this does not mean that IVF should be stopped or even restricted. It does mean, however, that we need to temper our enthusiasm for new treatments because they seem to represent a panacea.

HOW MUCH DOES IT ALL COST?

Most IVF in Britain is private; only a very few units are even partly funded by the National Health Service. IVF may be available in a few teaching hospitals on a semi-private basis. The money charged by these units often goes to help patients who cannot afford private fees and to pay for research. Without research, IVF will never improve, and because of this these units are often very deserving of private fees and support. It is regrettable that, too often, couples are prepared to pay for IVF at private clinics until their money runs out, and then come to these very hard-pressed academic units expecting further treatment. This is a pity because, apart from anything else, it is largely the academic units with their policy of ploughing back private fees which are mainly contributing to progress in improving IVF treatments.

HOW TO CHOOSE AN IVF CLINIC

Once the decision to have IVF has been made, there is the difficulty of choosing a good IVF clinic. There are several ways to get information, none of which is always satisfactory. They include:

● *Referral by a family doctor or a gynaecologist at a local hospital.* Some people rely on what their GPs or their gynaecologist tell them. Sadly, many family doctors and, incidentally, very many consultant gyanecologists do not thoroughly check the IVF clinics they recommend. They usually have very little experience of IVF and may actually be in a worse position than the couple to make a proper decision. Whilst a doctor's referral is best, our profession undoubtedly needs to try harder to get really accurate information about suitable IVF clinics so that patients have the best choice.

● *The media.* Some people are heavily influenced by what they read in the press, but they are quite often wrong to be so. For example, the *Independent*, normally an excellent newspaper, has, in the past, published a list of British IVF clinics with the services each offers; moreover, this guide includes data on success rates, which normally you might think was the best yardstick of all. Unfortunately, claimed success rates are not always verifiable. A clinic which is not very successful, and which relies on its income from private practice, is hardly likely to publish success rates which are less good than those of its competitors. This has been pointed out in the medical press in an honest and impressive letter by one of Britain's most respected IVF scientists, Dr Simon Fishel from Nottingham. His contentions are borne out by the fact that some success rates claimed in the aforementioned survey look rather better on paper than in practice. This is why at least one leading responsible clinic has refused to advertise in this newspaper's survey. Press reports are definitely the worst way to get accurate information about any IVF clinic.

● *Self-help or counselling organisations.* The two best organisations in Britain are CHILD and ISSUE (*see* pp. 348 and 349), both of which run excellent nationwide networks which provide advice and information including a list of IVF clinics. Inevitably, the information in this list is based entirely on what they had been *told* by the clinics, but at least they have sufficient experience to be wary of the exaggerated claims which can surround some work in this field.

None of these three alternatives is ideal by any means. If I were in need of IVF, there would be certain points about which I would like reassurance before committing myself to a particular clinic. For what they are worth, here are some of them:

● Did we like and feel confident with the team of doctors and nurses we met there? Did they seem like a team? Do they get on with each other?

● Do patients see a doctor regularly at most visits, rather than a member of the paramedical staff? Do patients tend to see the same individuals during treatment, ensuring proper continuity of care? Good units try to ensure good continuity and communication because so many patients are otherwise confused by conflicting information.

● Before treatment, does the clinic carry out adequate tests to establish the diagnosis as precisely as possible? This may seem impossible for a lay person to decide, but it is fairly simple to find out whether they bother to take a uterine X-ray (hysterosalpingogram, or HSG) when needed, or examine personally X-rays taken earlier at another hospital. Do they also do other ancillary tests, such as hormone tests, scans or a post-coital test, before committing you to IVF?

● Do they have an independent counsellor offering a free service available for your special problems? By 'independent' I mean not someone on the medical staff who is involved in the actual treatments. An independent counsellor can stand outside your treatment and help you focus on what may be best for you and your partner.

● Do they offer only IVF, or are all infertility treatments properly done? Clinics which focus on IVF as their sole or main treatment tend to offer this to the exclusion of other treatments. This is convenient for them, but may not be in your best interests.

● Who do you know who got pregnant there? This may seem a remarkably silly question, but in the United States, there are over 260 IVF clinics and nearly half of them have yet to produce a baby!

● Who do you know who failed treatment there? Were they satisfied with what they were told and how treatment generally went?

● How much monitoring of the treatment cycle is done routinely? Generally speaking, clinics which do regular hormone tests tend to get somewhat better results; they also have a better idea of what has gone wrong if the treatment fails.

● Is there just one fixed drug régime for getting the woman to produce many eggs, or do they tailor the treatment to suit her body and circumstances? On the whole, programmes with fixed régimes get less good results.

● Do they do very careful, repeated assessments of sperm quality before the IVF attempt? A good unit will have a set of precisely worked-out values for sperm quality, and will cancel an attempt early if they feel that there is really no chance of fertilisation. This is really very important because it is far too easy to try IVF when the attempt is doomed to failure.

● Can they do egg collections (or other treatments) at weekends?

● Do you have a choice of local or general anaesthesia and is an anaesthetist invariably present during your egg collection to ensure your safety?

● Do they do egg collection by both laparoscopy and ultrasound?

● Do their scientists examine all the eggs eighteen hours after mixing them with the sperm? This step is essential to ensure that a dividing egg has actually fertilised (*see* p. 207).

● How many embryos do they routinely put back into the uterus? In general, less good clinics need to transfer more embryos to produce pregnancy rates which approach the results of the better clinics. This is important because the more embryos that are transferred, the greater the risk of multiple birth, miscarriage, and premature delivery.

● How much do they charge? If they are charging much more

than other clinics – say, over £1,700 (excluding the cost of drugs[33]) – they may be overcharging. If they are charging much less – say, much under £1,000 – they are almost certainly not offering the most effective treatment. To some extent, you get what you pay for – cut-price IVF clinics may offer cut-price treatment.

● If the treatment fails, will you be able to see the director of the clinic personally? In good clinics, the director should be available (by appointment) to see couples who have failed their treatment cycle.[34] He should be able to go through your treatment cycle with you both, working out what, if anything, went wrong, where improvements might be made and whether a further IVF attempt or other treatment is justified.

ASSESSMENT OF A CLINIC'S RESULTS

One of the most difficult things when choosing an IVF clinic is assessing its performance. Nobody in their right mind would choose a clinic which gets inconsistent results, or which has a higher than average failure rate. Although there is always pressure on clinics to announce their results to patients, pride and commercial considerations may lead an IVF clinic to give 'results' tinged with unjustified optimism. Prospective clients must be very careful in assessing figures which are given out, because there are many ways in which results can be made to look better than they really are.

---

[33] The cost of the drugs is an important issue which needs urgent attention. I have only recently discovered that many chemists, and quite a few hospitals, mark up the cost of these drugs very considerably, so much so that couples can spend £200 or even £300 extra over the basic retail price. This unfair practice should be halted, possibly by clinics selling the drugs themselves at the basic cost price. We intend to institute this approach in our own service.

[34] I should add that whether you are a paying or free patient, this kind of follow-up appointment should, in my view, be offered free of charge. This is information and time for which you have already paid heavily. Some clinics are perfectly happy to see the patient who failed for further consultation, but at a price. This is iniquitous, and sensible couples would do well to avoid such establishments.

Pregnancy rates and therefore measurements of success can be expressed in many differing ways:

METHOD OF ASSESSMENT	AVERAGE IN UK CLINICS %	CURRENTLY BEST RESULTS %	WORST %
1. Pregnancy per embryo transfer	24.5	37	0
2. Pregnancy per egg collection	20.4	33	0
3. Pregnancy per stimulated cycle	17.3	29	0
4. Pregnancy per cycle started	No statistics available	Not available	0
5. Live births per transfer	17.6	28	0
6. Live births per egg collection	14.7	24	0
7. Live births per stimulated cycle	12.5	23	0
8. Live births per cycle started	No statistics available	Not available	0

Here, then, are no fewer than eight different measurements of success. These figures should certainly make you think, because they are taken from the official statistics of the Government's own body, the HFEA. Some clinics have had no success at all. It is simply not good enough for a clinic to claim over a 30 per cent success rate, as so many do, because this live birth rate has never been achieved. Pregnancy is very different from live births. No patients attending such a clinic merely want pregnancy – they want a baby. Some clinics have a much higher miscarriage rate than others and some more ectopics, hence the discrepancy. Moreover, IVF is like a gigantic hurdle race; there are many stages at which the participants can fall flat on their face. It is possible for a cycle to be started, but abandoned because the conditions or response to initial drug treatment are inadequate. Centres which prudently abandon impropitious cycles early on in larger numbers will appear to have a better than average success if they only report completed treatments. Obviously, results per embryo transfer will also invariably seem better, because so many patients don't produce eggs, or fertilise them, or because their embryos do not develop properly.

If you are considering IVF and think this is muddling, or even possibly threatening, the situation is actually even more complicated than this. Success rates claimed by clinics also depend very largely on other factors which need to be taken into account, if one is to make sensible choices about where to be treated:

● *Number of embryos transferred per patient.* Clinics needing to transfer three or four embryos in order to get a satisfactory pregnancy rate are not doing as good a job as clinics only transferring two embryos.

● *Average age of patients being treated.* Clinics treating younger women will always do better than those who are taking on the more difficult and less successful treatment of older women. Very few clinics state the average age of their clientèle, but they should be encouraged to do so in the interests of truth. A clinic treating women of an average age of thirty-three should do substantially better than those treating women with an average age of even two years older, say, thirty-five. Prospective patients should ask for this information; if it is not available, think carefully, because lack of this information suggests a poorly audited clinic.

● *Cause of infertility.* Patients with tubal disease only have a better chance of success than those with more than one cause for infertility, or couples with uterine problems or pure unexplained infertility. Patients have a right to know what the success rate is for their category.

● *Severity of disease.* A good example is the treatment of the male factor. Very frequently, very exaggerated claims are made for the success of treatment of male infertility. Success actually largely depends on the quality of the sperm the man produces, the numbers of sperm and their motility. Clinics treating male problems where the sperm are only marginally poor will do very substantially better. To make matters worse, measurements and assessment of sperm in different clinics varies hugely, and this also makes assessment of their results very difficult.

● *Previous failed IVF.* Centres that regularly accept patients who have previously failed IVF are taking on the 'hard cases'. An apparently lower success rate may just be justified if a clinic is trying to tackle large numbers of couples with very complex infertility problems.

● *Numbers of patients treated by that clinic.* Many clinics treat only a few patients and may, as often happens, have struck lucky with their first carefully selected treatments. This can give a very biased view of their success; for example, a clinic treating ten patients, of whom four get pregnant, could claim 40 per cent success. It is therefore important to ask how many patients are responsible for the success rate claimed.

SUCCESS AFTER EMBRYO FREEZING

If you think the above is confusing, consider the problem of assessing success when the option of embryo freezing is also included. For an example, look at these figures published and handed to patients from a typically good clinic (a clinic which I shall not name but which is one of the best at freezing). At first glance the results look very encouraging:

	1989	1990	1991	TOTAL
Frozen embryo transfers	81	133	138	352
Pregnancies	18	23	27	68
Pregnancy rate per transfer	22.2%	17.3%	19.6%	19.3%

These figures, compelling at first, because they suggest a sucess rate not so much worse than fresh embryo transfer in some clinics, do not tell the whole story. First, these figures do not take into account the number of embryos which, when frozen, did not thaw satisfactorily and therefore could not be transfered. This often happens as a huge proportion of frozen embryos are simply unsuitable for transfer after thawing, because they are damaged. Failure to give these statistics gives patients an unreasonably rosy view of the likelihood of their frozen embryos giving rise to a pregnancy. Second, these figures take no account of the miscarriage rate after frozen embryo storage, which tends to be high. Nor, of course, are the number of live births recorded, nor the numbers of embryos transferred simultaneously in order to get a pregnancy.

GIFT

GIFT – gamete intrafallopian transfer – is newer than IVF. Eggs are taken from the ovaries and mixed with sperm, and they are immediately placed in the Fallopian tube of the woman, before fertilisation. It is different from IVF because the embryo is not formed outside the body; instead, the egg is fertilised in its natural environment.

The invention of GIFT should be credited to Dr Tesarik and his colleagues in Czechoslovakia, whose idea it first was. This team transferred egg and sperm into the Fallopian tube of a woman undergoing tubal surgery in 1983. About a year or so later, Dr Ricardo Asch, working in San Antonio, Texas, reported a pregnancy following this manoeuvre. Perhaps slightly unreasonably, Dr Asch has collected most credit for the invention of tubal egg transfer. Following heavy promotion, GIFT has since become very popular, particularly in the United States, because it does not require sophisticated laboratory equipment for embryo culture.

GIFT is different from IVF, though there are similarities. An embryo is not formed in culture, but in the woman's own tubal fluid. This was thought to be an advantage as the precise needs of a developing human embryo are not fully understood. We are unable to mimic the ideal environment for fertilised eggs in the laboratory. GIFT overcomes this problem because eggs and sperm are put straight back into their natural environment. This means, of course, that the tube is not bypassed during GIFT treatment – another difference from IVF – and as a result, GIFT is not a useful treatment when tubal disease is the indication for treatment. GIFT also works best when more than one egg is collected and placed with the sperm. Like IVF, the woman needs drug treatment to stimulate the ovaries to produce several eggs simultaneously. The eggs are usually collected by laparoscopy, rather than by ultrasound, because the laparoscope is needed to guide the surgeon when the eggs and sperm are being placed in the Fallopian tube.

WHEN IS GIFT INDICATED?

The main reason for GIFT treatment is when no cause for the infertility has been found. It may also be used when there is a problem with the cervical mucus and post-coital tests are always negative. I wrote, in the first edition of this book, that 'high success rates are claimed for GIFT by many clinics, but at the best centres, there is no evidence that the results are any better than those for IVF.' I have come under considerable criticism by my colleagues for this statement, but it is now clear that GIFT is not as good as IVF, if the IVF is done using good laboratory methods in an experienced centre.

WHY IS GIFT NOT A PARTICULARLY
SATISFACTORY TREATMENT?

Of course, GIFT quite often works. Some happy parents can testify to this. However, it is not as satisfactory as good IVF, and this is some of the evidence:
● Most couples having GIFT treatment are, except for their undiagnosed inability to conceive, normal. They undergo a very complex and expensive treatment when there is nothing demonstrably wrong. Quite often, much simpler treatments would be as effective.
● Until recently there had been no proper trials of GIFT, comparing it with other simpler treatments nor, indeed, with IVF. A recent, controlled trial at Hammersmith Hospital has now been completed for those with genuinely unexplained infertility (where all known causes have been carefully and meticulously excluded first). After three cycles of GIFT, spaced

at regular intervals of one year, 52 per cent of patients had a pregnancy; after three cycles of IVF over one year 84 per cent of comparable patients conceived successfully.

● Many woman are coerced into GIFT by their own desperation. They often feel that they get inadequate testing and treatment, and expect that this treatment will answer their problem. Many women who have failed GIFT treatment have subsequently conceived with simpler and cheaper remedies.

● GIFT treatment involves the return of eggs and sperm into the body *before* fertilisation. This means that less diagnostic information is obtained than with IVF. With the latter, the couple learn that they can produce an embryo. We have already seen that many eggs do not fertilise, or when fertilised, do not develop into embryos which are capable of subsequent implantation and normal pregnancy. It stands to reason that it is better to put embryos back into the uterus which have already been observed under a microscope to be healthy and developing, rather than to place unfertilised eggs into the tube in mere hope.

● GIFT usually involves laparoscopy. IVF can now be done with ultrasound alone, avoiding the need for a general anaesthetic.

● In Britain, GIFT is being increasingly used in district general hospitals which do not have adequate facilities and do not provide comprehensive treatment. It has also been 'pushed' very hard by one drug company which has a vested interest in selling expensive fertility drugs. This use of GIFT is detrimental to fertility treatments as a whole because it diverts attention from more important, cheaper treatments, and squanders precious NHS resources.

GIFT is being very widely used for male infertility. The rationale is that, by placing the sperm and egg very close together, there may be more chance of fertilisation. A major disadvantage of GIFT is that, unlike IVF, we are not able to check to see whether the sperm have fertilised the eggs and have functioned normally. I have quite serious misgivings about GIFT in such instances. We do not know why it works, nor even how well it works. It is not clear whether it is the preparation of the sperm, or the mixing of the sperm directly with the egg, or the timed stimulation of ovulation which really produces the increase in pregnancies which is claimed.[35]

ZIFT, T-SET, PROST, POST, DIPI, TUFT, DOT, VEST AND SHIFT

Some infertility clinics are not happy unless they have coined their own acronym. These terms have two things in common – each has been coined by someone eager (often without any justification whatsoever beyond an ability to spell four-letter words) to be at the forefront of the medical practice of IVF, and none of the procedures they represent has any really proven value. In case you still want to know, these terms are:

ZIFT: Zygote Intra-Fallopian Transfer. The embryo is transferred directly to the Fallopian tube, usually using a laparoscope.

T-SET: Tubal Sperm and Egg Transfer. Coined by a particular practitioner presumably too stubborn or conceited to use the perfectly acceptable term GIFT.

PROST: A Pronuclear Oocyte (an embryo in the earliest stage of development) is transferred to the Fallopian tube.

POST: Peritoneal Oocyte and Sperm Transfer. In this treatment, eggs and sperm are injected directly into the abdominal cavity, in the hope that the Fallopian tube will pick up any resulting embryo.

DIPI: Direct Intra-Peritoneal Sperm Injection. Sperm are injected through the vaginal wall, directly into the abdomen.

TUFT: Transuterine Fallopian Transfer. A mixture of sperm and eggs is loaded into a fine catheter, introduced through

---

[35] I have inflamed some of my colleagues by suggesting that GIFT is 'one of the greatest confidence tricks that has been perpetrated'. I admit that this phrase was a bit 'over the top', but this is an expensive treatment, of unproved efficacy, which could always be replaced by IVF to considerable advantage both in terms of success and diagnostic value, providing units concentrated more on improving the IVF facilities. What I meant was that it is wasteful for NHS resources not to be devoted to the best treatment.

the vagina and hence into one or other tube. An interesting example of man's ingenuity which does not appear to give any measurable benefit to woman.

DOT: Direct Oocyte Transfer (into the uterus). Two out of the original thirty-one patients conceived; should be renamed DOTTY.

VEST: Vaginal Egg and Sperm Transfer. Some centres have hit on the idea of bottling up the sperm and egg in a little tube and putting it temporarily in the woman's vagina, where it can be incubated. This saves on electricity bills.

SHIFT: Synchronised Hysteroscopic Intra-Fallopian Transfer. Sperm are transferred into the Fallopian tube via a hysteroscope inserted in the uterus. Professor Pat Taylor, from Canada, has waggishly suggested that the 'F' could easily be dropped from this acronym and Synchronised Hysteroscopic Intra-Fallopian Transfer would still remain just about as valuable.

CHAPTER TWELVE

Donor Insemination and Egg Donation

We have seen how inadequate the treatment of male infertility really is. Medical intervention makes a difference in few cases. If treatment fails and the man is proved sterile, there are basically three choices. First, a couple may come to terms with the problem, grieve the loss of childbearing and accept that they will never have children. Second, they may look into the possibility of adoption; unfortunately, this is extremely difficult in nearly all developed countries because there are very few 'unwanted' babies. The third alternative is donor insemination with sperm taken from another, fertile man. I emphasise that donor insemination is a *substitute* and *not* a treatment for infertility. A couple have to come to terms with their infertility before taking this decision.

Just as some infertile men produce no sperm at all (for which, of course, there is no treatment), some women have total ovarian failure – that is, their ovaries are quite incapable of producing eggs. While there is also no treatment for this uncommon condition, an option is for them to accept eggs donated from a fertile woman.

While donor insemination is technically relatively simple, treatment involving donated eggs is more complicated, requiring in vitro fertilisation. Although these treatments are essentially very different, they both raise similar medical, ethical and emotional issues.

Donor Insemination

Until recently, donor insemination was always referred to as 'Artificial Insemination by Donor', or AID. It has now had its name changed to avoid confusion with AIDS, or 'Acquired Immune Deficiency Syndrome'.

Donor insemination involves taking semen, produced by masturbation, from a fertile donor, who usually remains anonymous. This is then inseminated into the vagina and cervix of the woman, at a time in the menstrual cycle when she is judged to be fertile. Commonly, insemination is timed using ultrasound tests or blood tests, but a few clinics are now getting their clients to use the urinary LH dipstick (see p. 43). Unfortunately, many clinics use only unreliable temperature charting.

Good clinics usually inseminate on at least two occasions during any one cycle, to give a better chance of covering the fertile period. The insemination is done as described on pp. 208–9.

The main indication for using donor semen is male infertility. Most responsible doctors will not use donor sperm unless there is no chance of a pregnancy by other methods. Donor semen may also be suggested if the man is a carrier of a specific genetic disease; sperm from a donor free from that particular genetic abnormality allow a couple to have unaffected children.

SPERM DONORS

These are generally university students. I get the impression that, in the United States, medical students are regarded as ideal donors, which says a lot about the value judgements of the American medical profession.

In Professor Snowden's book *The Artificial Family* he describes the case of Addison Hard of Jefferson Medical College in Philadelphia. Dr Hard wrote to *Medical World* in 1909 claiming to have been involved in the first case of donor insemination in 1884. A local merchant who was sterile had married a woman ten years younger. The case was discussed in the medical school with the students, of whom one was Addison Hard. The students agreed that semen should be obtained from 'the best-looking member of the class' and then inseminated. Hard maintains that this was done while the wife was anaesthetised and that neither the merchant nor his spouse knew about it. After the woman conceived, the merchant was informed but pleaded that his pregnant wife should not be told. The surgeon in charge went to his grave with the secret, but when the merchant's son was twenty-five years old he was visited by the excessively handsome Dr Hard, who could not resist publishing his experiences.

Donors are screened as carefully as possible for serious illness and infection, and they are normally free from any genetic disease. Attempts are usually made to match the donor's physical characteristics with those of the woman's partner. Height, build, colour of hair, complexion and eyes are recorded and matched as closely as possible, as are ethnic group and religion if requested. Most centres ensure that the blood group of the donor is also matched to the couple, so that there will be no risk of the baby developing Rhesus disease.

A second important feature about donors is that they are rarely of proven fertility. Most have never had children nor, indeed, are they in long-term relationships. (If they were, they probably would be much less likely to give their semen because they would begin to understand the implications of giving their genetic material to a third party in this way.) If repeated inseminations with one particular donor's semen fail to produce a pregnancy, most clinics switch to a different donor. Unfortunately, most donor programmes have a limited number of good fertile donors (especially since the appearance of AIDS) and this inevitably means that semen from one donor is often used for a large number of pregnancies. This has obvious serious disadvantages. Above all, it increases the risk of two people (both children conceived via donor insemination and therefore both related) meeting in future and having children of their own.

This, above all, worries very many religious people. It also has important genetic implications as inbreeding greatly increases the risk of genetic abnormalities in the population.

Donors are virtually always anonymous. This is partly to protect the donor, and partly for the benefit of the recipient. A donor does not want any responsibility for the offspring. There is growing concern about this because, in Britain, it has become widely felt that the children born following donor insemination should know who their genetic fathers are. The law at present is very unsatisfactory. Most donors would not be prepared to donate if they had to identify themselves; it has therefore been suggested that the insemination clinics keep non-identifying information about the donors, so that children can at least have some rough idea of what sort of people their real fathers are. This may also be very important if, for example, the child develops a genetic disease later in life thought to be inherited from the father.

What is very clear is that donors are not properly counselled or even advised about the implications of what they are doing. Donors are usually young, with no ties, and may not fully recognise how they may feel in future about having donated sperm. It is said that many donors, years after donation and perhaps following marriage, worry deeply about their uncertainty as to whether they have children whom they do not know and for whom they can take no responsibility.

Until recently a child born following donor insemination was illegitimate and the so-called 'father' had no legal rights. This anomaly in British law was rectified by parliament in the Family Law Reform Act of 1988. The birth certificate may now be signed by the 'father' and the child is legitimately his.

OBTAINING DONOR SEMEN

Opinions vary about whether donors should be paid. This certainly introduces a commercial element, with the inevitable risk that an unhealthy donor may be persuaded to sell his semen, perhaps passing on a serious infection. Donors who give away their semen are certainly altruistic, but this kind of altruism is increasingly rare in our society – particularly with the tests and inconvenience a donor experiences. A rather poor compromise is usually reached whereby the donor is paid his 'expenses' only.

ETHNIC AND RELIGIOUS ISSUES

One difficulty that most clinics have is finding a donor with a specific racial or ethnic background. For example, Asian donors are very difficult to find: few Indians in Britain, for example, will consider donating sperm; and similar difficulties are experienced in getting Chinese donors. This can be very difficult for a couple who are eager to accept donor insemination, but want very much to preserve their own racial and cultural identity.

INSEMINATION WITH THE SEMEN OF A KNOWN DONOR

Some couples much prefer to be inseminated with the sperm of a person whom they know. Usually this is a close relative, but occasionally it may be a particular friend. Most medical practitioners are very wary of this as it creates the potential of a new type of family relationship. For one thing, there is always the risk of the donor watching his child grow up under parental guidance of which he disapproves. He may feel very possessive towards the child and attempt to interfere in later life with his or her care or psychological well-being. Such arrangements may also tend to create an unhealthy bond between the donor and the mother. Such a bond could destroy a marital relationship. The other problem is that a child perceives that he or she has, in effect, three parents. This could be very disruptive for the child's proper development, and could cause great distress if he or she felt unhappy with various parental decisions. It is likely that the brunt of these problems would be worst at puberty, when a child needs a stable nuclear family.[36]

[36] Although I am extremely nervous about 'known or related donors', I have inseminated three couples where the donor was a member of the family. On each occasion my decision was accompanied by great soul-searching, and very reluctantly taken. Five children have been born to these families; the oldest is now fifteen. One family are great personal friends, so I have had

SHOULD WE CONSIDER DONOR INSEMINATION?

The decision to have donor insemination is a very personal one, and nobody can tell you whether or not it is right for your relationship. It is like adoption in many ways, with the advantage that the child will be genetically related to at least one of you. Moreover, donor insemination is much easier to achieve. It is said that, every year, there are well over 10,000 babies born following donor insemination in both the United Kingdom and the USA.

There is something of a stigma associated with donor insemination. Many men are remarkably reluctant to admit that they are sterile, and so they and their partners keep the insemination a closely guarded secret. Friends and even parents – the prospective grandparents – are not told. Certainly, whether you are going to reveal the true origins of your child is something you need to think over very carefully. It is wise, indeed probably essential, to go for professional counselling. There are a number of hospitals and clinics which provide this, and it is also available in the private sector.

QUESTIONS THAT MAY BE ASKED

WILL MY PARTNER LOVE A CHILD FROM A SPERM DONOR?

Women sometimes ask this question, but in my experience, this is not a problem. The male partner becomes deeply involved and shares pregnancy and birth. I have seen so many husbands in this situation made obviously and rapturously happy that I cannot believe that there is a serious risk of estrangement. If the decision is taken mutually and it is freely discussed, the man's

---

opportunity to observe closely the result of my decision . I am glad to say that in all the cases where I have been involved the outcome, so far, has been entirely happy.

relationship with the child should be just the same as that of other children with their genetic fathers. The environment in which we bring up children is, in many ways, much more important for their development than a blood relationship. Women can be assured that their child will rapidly take on the characteristics and outlook of their partner[37] and he will be just as involved in being a parent.

Most experts who have studied this aspect of donor insemination find no evidence of any particular problems – either emotional or psychological – within marriages where donor sperm have been used. Dr Margaret Jackson, a remarkably brave and intelligent woman who was perhaps the great British pioneer of donor insemination, felt that, in her experience (which was greater than that of anyone else I know), marriages where donor semen was used were frequently enriched and improved.

Dr Robert Snowden, eminent professor of sociology in Exeter and a leading expert in this field, who is properly very cautious about donor insemination, agrees that there is evidence to suggest continued bonding between the children and their 'fathers'. Even when a donor insemination marriage fails, there is good evidence that the husbands often feel the same way about the children and wish to care for them as if they were genetically their own.

It is worth remembering that there are many fathers who are genetically related to their children who treat them appallingly. A genetic relationship is no guarantee of family harmony.

WILL MY CHILD LOVE HIS/HER FATHER?

Everything I know about donor insemination leads me to conclude that children regard 'adoptive' fathers as theirs. Many children in this situation seem to regard their parents particularly

[37] One woman I know has been repeatedly told that her donor insemination child 'looks much more like her husband's family' than her own. Apparently, this is a very common experience.

highly, because they went through so much to have them. One boy, having had things explained, wrote: 'He's my Daddy – I'm just pleased that they loved me enough to be able to share their secret with me and with my sister. I feel tremendous warm love for them both . . .'

HOW TO GET DONOR INSEMINATION

People sometimes find that their doctor may well be reluctant to raise the subject at all and that they may need to ask whether this could be considered. Donor insemination in Britain is mostly available only privately. There are only eleven clinics in Britain that I know of which offer donor insemination on a National Health Service basis; this is not many when you consider that there are 200 health districts in England and Wales and these few clinics may well be geographically out of reach. Private treatments are not cheap, and are certainly expensive if proper ovulation monitoring is carried out as well. Some clinics screen the recipients very inadequately, even though their donors are properly monitored.

ISSUE (see p. 349) can put prospective couples in touch with reliable donor cinics. The Family Planning Association may be able to offer advice about what is available in your area. It is worth remembering, incidentally, that most clinics, even the private ones, have waiting lists for insemination.

When going for donor insemination, one should remember that this is not nearly as successful as natural intercourse. Usually no more than 50 per cent of women will be pregnant after nine treatments; this means considerable upheaval and expense. It is also worth keeping in mind that donor insemination is not very pleasant emotionally; some women find it very clinical, and, unfortunately, the burden of the treatment is something they cannot easily share with their partners, who are left out by the very nature of what is being done.

One word of advice: if you do go to a private clinic for donor insemination, do not have endless repeated treatments without getting yourself checked. If there is no pregnancy within four or five months of trying insemination, it is important to make certain that any fertility tests that have not been done are completed.

AN UNUSUAL CASE OF DONOR INSEMINATION

Artificial insemination is not so very new. One of the earliest pregnancies achieved was reported in the *Lancet* over 100 years ago, in January 1875.

Dr Capers, an army surgeon, fought with General Ulysses Grant in the American Civil War. In May 1863 a comrade-in-arms, next to whom he stood in the line of battle, fell to the earth with a wound from a minnie bullet. Almost simultaneously, Dr Capers heard a piercing scream from a house 150 yards behind. Examining the young man, he found a fracture of the leg, but the bullet had 'ricocheted from these lower parts, and, in its onward flight, had passed through the scrotum, carrying off the left testicle'. Dr Capers dressed the wounds, and minutes later 'the esteemable matron of the house' ran up in the greatest distress saying that her seventeen-year-old daughter had been badly wounded a few minutes earlier. He ran to the house to find that she, too, had a bullet wound in her lower abdomen. He attended her but thought she would die. The army was forced to retreat; fortunately, the girl recovered and the doctor rejoined his regiment.

Six months later, the fortunes of war found Dr Capers back in the same place. He visited his young patient, who 'was in excellent health and spirits, but her abdomen was enormously enlarged, so much so as to resemble pregnancy at the seventh or eighth month . . . Just 278 days from the date of the receipt of the wound, I delivered this young lady of a fine boy weighing eight pounds – imagine the surprise and mortification of the entire family which may be better imagined than described. Although I found the hymen intact before delivery, I gave no credence to the earnest and oft-repeated assertions of the young lady about her innocence and her purity.'

Three weeks later, Dr Capers was called to see the child. The grandmother insisted 'there was something wrong about the genitals'. Dr Capers found a swelling in the scrotum of the baby which he immediately extracted; this swelling turned out to be a musket bullet, of the type used by the Confederate Army, battered but intact. 'Picture my astonishment,' says Dr Capers, 'but there can be no other solution to the phenomenon.' He explained the situation to the family and to his soldier friend who 'at first, most naturally, appeared skeptical, but concluded to visit the mother.' Three months later, they married and later had three more children. Dr Capers was later to observe that none of the children so closely resembled their father 'as the first one'.

Egg donation

Egg donation has only been possible since IVF and GIFT have become established. In this treatment, the sperm of the male partner is used to fertilise eggs from a female donor. The embryos which are produced are transferred to the uterus of the infertile woman, where they grow normally. Unlike donor insemination, egg donation has the advantage that both partners are involved in any resulting pregnancy. Even though the infertile woman does not contribute genetically to her own child, she carries it within her own body and she gives birth to it.

WHAT ARE THE INDICATIONS FOR EGG DONATION?

Egg donation is almost exclusively used to treat women whose own ovaries are not producing any eggs. The main indication is therefore primary ovarian failure (or premature menopause). A small percentage of women stop menstruating and enter their menopause much earlier in life than normal.

In very rare cases, egg donation may also be suitable for a few other conditions. These include:

● Women whose own eggs repeatedly fail to fertilise during IVF treatments. The presumption is that there is an inherent abnormality of the eggs which prevents fertilisation. A few units are now recommending that such women consider having eggs from a donor.

● Women whose ovaries respond very badly to drug therapy to increase ovulation during IVF treatment and from whom eggs cannot be collected due to scar tissue or ovarian cyst formation. Severe endometriosis of the ovaries is one such indication. Most of these women have had extensive pelvic inflammatory disease which has severely damaged both tubes and both ovaries.

● Women without any ovarian tissue, such as those with Turner's syndrome, a congenital disease which is caused by a woman having only one X-chromosome instead of two. Turner's syndrome results in absent periods, poor breast and genital development, and shortness of stature; a few sufferers also have heart problems. All are subfertile.

● Women who are carriers of severe genetic diseases which may cause their children to die or suffer greatly. These women may also request egg donation which, of course, allows them to have perfectly healthy children.

HOW IS EGG DONATION DONE?

Women who are in need of donor eggs are not normally having periods. This means that the lining of the uterus – the endometrium – is very thin and inadequate. Even if an embryo were placed there, implantation could not happen because of the inadequacy of the uterine environment. For egg donation to be successful, it first is necessary to stimulate the uterus with hormones. This is done by giving the hormones oestrogen and progesterone in a cyclical fashion, usually for about three months, creating artificial menstrual cycles. At the end of this time, donated eggs can be fertilised in the laboratory with the partner's sperm and resulting embryos can be transferred to the artificially stimulated uterus. This has a very good chance of success.

Alternatively, GIFT can be done (*see* p. 235). The uterus is stimulated by hormone therapy in the same way, and once an artificial menstrual cycle has been established, eggs and sperm are placed in a Fallopian tube using a laparoscope.

Egg donation treatment may actually be more difficult if a woman is having regular menstrual cycles, because the periods may require suppression, so that the embryos can be placed in the uterus at the time when they are most likely to implant. Women with Turner's syndrome are even more difficult to treat because they have had a major hormone deficiency since birth. Because they have no ovarian tissue at all, they have never made much oestrogen. This usually results in the uterus being less well developed than normal, and makes an embryo transfer less likely to succeed.

WHAT PROBLEMS MIGHT BE ENCOUNTERED?

There is, as yet, very little hard information about the problems a recipient of donor eggs may experience. It is a new field, and unlike donor insemination, which has been carried out routinely for at least forty years, there has been only a tiny number of babies born via egg donation. The general feeling is that the problems may be rather similar to those experienced with donor insemination. However, women who receive donated eggs play a much more active biological role than do infertile men whose partners undergo donor insemination. This may mean that egg donation will probably be attended with rather less psychological risk.

EGG DONORS

Egg donors are not easy to come by. Many IVF clinics use spare eggs gleaned from women undergoing IVF treatment. IVF results in the production of many eggs simultaneously, many of which will not be needed for the patient's treatment. The rest of the eggs are surplus to requirements. Thus, for example, if patient A produces twenty eggs during an IVF cycle, a few of these eggs would be set aside for fertilisation by sperm from the male partner of patient B, who is awaiting egg donation.

All this sounds very well, but to my mind there are very severe ethical and medical drawbacks. Supposing that, of the twenty eggs obtained, fifteen are reserved for patient A's own treatment and the remaining five are given to B? There is always the real possibility that none of the eggs allocated for patient A's treatment will fertilise; alternatively, none of the embryos transferred to patient A's uterus may result in a pregnancy. Meanwhile, patient B might have got pregnant with patient A's eggs. The donor is, in effect, disadvantaged by her donation, for had she received the eggs that B received, she might have become pregnant. When you consider that A may have waited a long time for the treatment, or paid a large sum for it, she clearly has had a very poor deal. In spite of this problem, by far the more common source of donor eggs at present is patients undergoing IVF treatment. Why is this? Alternative donors to IVF patients also present difficulties. Sperm donation is physically very easy; indeed, some would suggest pleasurable. Egg donation is very different. To collect eggs, a minor operation is needed – either laparoscopy or ultrasound needle collection through the vagina – and a general anaesthetic may be required. These procedures carry real risks, quite acceptable if a woman needs treatment but not so acceptable if she is gaining no possible benefit from the procedure. As if the risk of egg collection were not enough, there is the problem of ovarian stimulation. To get eggs, treatment with daily fertility injections is required. This also carries risks, mainly that of over-stimulating the ovaries and causing cysts. Sometimes this complication requires hospital treatment. Moreover, fertility drugs require fairly intensive monitoring with daily ultrasound and blood tests – at the very least, a severe inconvenience for a working woman or one with a young family.

Some clinics try to overcome these difficulties by encouraging an infertile woman's friends or relatives to come forward to give eggs. I believe that this is fraught with danger. We have already seen why having a related sperm donor may cause innumerable problems to a child or its parents later in life. These problems are likely to be very similar for egg donation. Indeed, they may be even greater because of the amount of effort and commitment an egg donor needs to have to go through with her donation. She may well feel very possessive about any child that results and may take more than a dispassionate interest in his or her subsequent welfare and well-being.

For these reasons, some clinics have decided that the only logical and ethically acceptable way of obtaining donor eggs is to collect them when women come into hospital for other gynaecological procedures, such as hysterectomy or sterilisation. This does not solve the ethical problems of the complications from fertility drugs, but does remove the need for a special anaesthetic or surgical procedure to collect eggs. Moreover, such women are generally strongly motivated to help others, very often having seen the suffering that infertility brings. Alternatively, they have had the pleasure of bringing up a family and want to give something to those who have not had this experience. Those coming in for sterilisation also are usually quite fertile, producing eggs of good quality, hence the request for sterilisation. The problem with using gynaecological patients is that of age. Most women having sterilisation or hysterectomy are close to or over forty years old. By the age of forty, most women are producing a very large proportion of abnormal eggs (*see* p. 87). It cannot be ethical to transfer defective eggs to an infertile patient, knowing that she stands a high risk of giving birth to a genetically defective baby – especially when that genetic defect has not been engendered by her own ovaries.

Embryo donation

In recent years a number of frozen embryos, stored after successful IVF treatment, have been preserved in liquid nitrogen banks. If the genetic parents have no further need of them, and if they wish, these embryos may be given away. Depending on their wishes, disposal may be simply thawing and destruction, or possibly donation for research purposes. Another alternative is to allow these embryos to be given to infertile couples who, for various reasons, have been totally unsuccessful at IVF. Embryo donation has been described as a form of 'adoption in utero'. It does have the clear advantage that the recipient does at least have the chance of giving birth to her 'adopted' child and nurturing it from the beginning of life. To date, there have been relatively few cases of successful embryo donation, but there is likely to be an increase in this treatment as more spare frozen embryos become available.

Telling the truth

One of the biggest criticisms of both egg, sperm and embryo donation is that they can both carry more than an element of deceit. To protect their children, and to cover up what is an area of shame and guilt for many couples, there is a strong desire to keep the facts of donor conception secret from everybody, including the children.

I am certain as I can be that such secrecy is completely misguided and wrong, and that it can build huge problems for the future. Family secrets have a habit of surfacing – usually at moments when the family is in crisis or following a severe quarrel. Imagine the consequences to children of finding out from one or other parent, in the middle of a heated quarrel or during a divorce, that they are not the offspring of their supposed fathers or mothers. A sudden rejection by, for example, a presumed father would be a very severe trauma indeed, and it may be impossible for a child to cope with this. Even in the most stable families, if the act of donor insemination is kept secret, there can be the most harmful, unforeseen circumstances.

Children conceived by donor insemination or donor eggs may be concerned to know who their genetic parents are. Most children in this situation simply want to confirm, if possible, that their genetic parents are well and healthy, but these feelings do not interfere with that of love felt for their own 'adopted' family unit. This, above all, is a good reason for openness.

Not infrequently, the attitude of secrecy is endorsed or fostered by the doctors doing the procedure. A classic example is the frequent use of mixed seminal specimens. Some practitioners, in order to give a couple the illusion that a child may be genetically their own, mix the semen of the infertile male partner with that of the donor. In this way, there is always the thought that the child might just possibly be the child of its 'adoptive' father, who may derive some benefit from this. I do not agree. If a couple needs the semen to be mixed, they are almost certainly not ready to consider donor insemination. To my mind, mixing semen specimens is simply compounding any problem that may arise after donor insemination. To be confused about the real parentage of one's own child is to confound the basis of family life.

HIV and AIDS

In recent years, there have been huge worries over the problems that AIDS creates. AIDS is a fatal disease, caused by the human immunodeficiency virus, or HIV, with which a prospective donor may be infected. This is an important concern with regard to both sperm and egg donation. Sperm donors are now screened to confirm that they are free of the virus. Moreover, their semen is held for a period of quarantine: all donor semen is frozen and stored in liquid nitrogen for a minimum of three months so that absence of the AIDS virus can be confirmed. This practice works to some extent against the infertile couple as semen that is frozen and then thawed is not quite as fertile as freshly ejaculated semen. However, it is an essential safeguard. (Some also worry that freezing the sperm may produce an abnormal child, but this is definitely not true.)

With eggs the situation is more complex. We saw in the previous chapter that freezing eggs is still very difficult, and carries dangers to the egg which may be made abnormal by freezing technology. Consequently donated eggs have to be transferred fresh to the uterus, which incurs the risk that dangerous viruses, such as HIV, may be carried over with the transferred eggs. One solution is to fertilise the donated egg first, then freeze the resulting embryo and hold it in quarantine for three or even six months. The donor is then retested to confirm absence of HIV. Only after that is the embryo transferred to the recipient's uterus. This is the safest course of action, but it does mean that that treatment process is dragged out over a long time. Also, the act of freezing embryos lowers their overall viability and results in a less good chance of pregnancy. Moreover, as discussed in the preceding chapter, egg freezing may just possibly carry certain long-term risks to the child which results.

PART THREE

PROBLEMS DURING EARLY PREGNANCY

CHAPTER THIRTEEN

Early Pregnancy Loss

Miscarriage

There are few events more distressing than a miscarriage, particularly after infertility treatment. This burden is inevitably borne by women, but it is sometimes forgotten how difficult it can be for the man to cope with this loss. It seems particularly harsh that women who may have been trying for years to get pregnant are rather more prone to miscarriage than others. If conception finally occurs after having endless investigations and years of fraught treatment, a miscarriage can bring complete despair.

We have already seen how infertile humans are. The early human embryo is very likely to fail to implant for a variety of different reasons. Some of the reasons are very obscure, and others very poorly understood by experts. If one does not know what is causing the problem, it is particularly hard to come to terms with it. Even when the embryo is implanted, early development may fail and no foetus may be formed. Worse still, late miscarriage – that is, loss of the pregnancy after the twelfth week – is quite common. Here we shall look at some of the reasons for this failure, and why early embryos are apparently so ill-protected by nature.

WHY IS MISCARRIAGE SO FREQUENT?

We do not know what proportion of embryos normally survive and become children. Actually, the only hard evidence we have about the frequency of miscarriage is from studying patients having IVF. Because embryos are deliberately placed into the uterus, it is relatively easy to work out how many women have a positive pregnancy test following this, and how many miscarry or end up with a live baby. For example, when we place a single embryo into the womb after fertilising it outside the body, there is about a 10 per cent chance of pregnancy. Unfortunately, figures from IVF treatment may not be completely reliable, because infertile women are prone to miscarry; IVF treatment itself may increase the chance of an early miscarriage.

Our solid information is therefore limited, but there is no other way of finding out precisely and accurately whether a normal woman has ovulated and, if so, whether the egg inside her body has fertilised. Knowledge from the study of natural menstrual cycles is circumstantial. We do know that, in an average month, a normal woman has a 12–20 per cent chance of getting pregnant (see p. 9). What we do not know is how often in her menstrual cycles she ovulates, or how often an egg becomes fertilised and, if so, how often it implants.

It has been calculated that, overall, about 23 per cent of human pregnancies are lost in the first five months. Many of these losses do occur very early, probably before the fourteenth day after conception, usually before a woman would even know she was pregnant, because, of course, menstruation does not generally start until fourteen days after ovulation. Such a very early pregnancy loss will seldom cause any symptoms.

HOW TO DETECT AN EARLY MISCARRIAGE

Most women who miscarry will have already felt pregnant, and usually will have had a delayed or absent period. However, a few who miscarry may be completely unaware that they were pregnant, and may not even have missed their period. Miscarriage may be heralded by one or two symptoms, or there may simply be a feeling that the pregnancy has ended.

VAGINAL BLEEDING

This is the most common symptom, and can occur at any time after a missed period. Quite often bleeding commences about six weeks after the last period. It is also said that the times of greatest risk are at eight, twelve and sixteen weeks – that is, at the times when a period would be expected if not pregnant. However, I don't believe this.

The bleeding may be quite light, not nearly as heavy as a menstrual period, or it can be very heavy indeed, with clots. On the whole, the more advanced the pregnancy, the more likely is heavy bleeding. Whatever the stage of pregnancy, if there is unexpected vaginal bleeding, it really is quite important to see the doctor immediately.

Bleeding during early pregnancy is extremely alarming and upsetting, and comes as an acute blow both to the woman and her partner. I remember when my wife had a relatively tiny amount of bleeding in early pregnancy, and I – a case-hardened gynaecologist, a miscarriage veteran – was surprised to find how very disturbed I felt. If you are a couple in this unfortunate situation, please remember that bleeding in very early pregnancy is extremely common. We find that, in almost 50 per cent of the pregnancies we monitor very closely at Hammersmith, following treatment in the infertility clinic, the women have some degree of vaginal bleeding, but very few actually abort.

The word 'abort' comes as a bit of a shock to some people. An 'abortion' is the medical term for any pregnancy lost before the twenty-eighth week (thereafter, it is called a 'stillbirth'). This term in no way implies that the pregnancy has been interfered with. Bleeding during early pregnancy is usually called a 'threatened abortion'. If the bleeding becomes very heavy and it is clear that the pregnancy has definitely been lost, it is generally referred to as an 'inevitable abortion'. I must emphasise, though, that even very heavy bleeding does not necessarily mean that the pregnancy has definitely been lost; on occasion I have seen women bleed profusely but keep their pregnancies. One thing is reassuring: no matter how heavy the bleeding, it will not damage a pregnancy if it survives. The bleeding cannot starve the baby of nutrients or oxygen.

Bleeding is usually much more obvious on going to the toilet. Very often, women rest in bed and the bleeding appears to stop, but as soon as they get up and walk about, and especially when they go to the toilet, they feel it all 'gushing away' from them. It is natural to think that, under these circumstances, going to the toilet or walking about has, in some way, encouraged the miscarriage to worsen. This is not true. What happens is that the blood continues to seep away, collecting at the top of the vagina; on rising, this all leaks away, often in large amounts. This is not an argument against the usefulness of bedrest. It certainly has a place in preventing miscarriage as the less one exercises and moves around the greater the blood flow to the pregnancy. I do think bedrest is quite sensible.

ABDOMINAL PAIN

Pain in the lower part of the abdomen is extremely common in pregnancy. I must strongly emphasise that only in very few cases does it mean that a miscarriage is threatened or, indeed, that there is anything necessarily wrong at all. None the less, crampy lower abdominal pain, especially if associated with some bleeding, strongly suggests miscarriage is imminent. The crampy pain is usually low down and is felt in the area just around or above the pubic bone. It may also be felt in the back, or at the top of the vagina. Some women describe it rather like labour pains.

Ectopic pregnancy (see p. 280) may present with quite similar symptoms. With miscarriage the bleeding usually starts first and pain commences afterwards; the reverse sometimes happens in ectopic pregnancy. Whatever the situation, if there are lower abdominal cramps or severe discomfort, the doctor should be contacted.

NOT FEELING PREGNANT ANY MORE

Some women, having felt very pregnant (perhaps with nausea and vomiting) suddenly stop feeling any symptoms. Now, before any pregnant woman reading this gets very upset, let me stress that it is extremely common to stop feeling pregnant during perfectly normal pregnancy. Nevertheless, a doctor's opinion may be worth while. A pregnancy test may be negative; an ultrasound scan may show lack of progress of the pregnancy.

WHY DO MISCARRIAGES HAPPEN?

Much of the time, the precise reason for a miscarriage is not clear. Why they are so common is a mystery. Those who have been unlucky enough to miscarry repeatedly should certainly do their best to find a reason. The following are the more common causes.

GENETIC ABNORMALITIES

An abnormal embryo is almost certainly the most common reason for miscarriage. Defective pregnancies are very common in humans; a miscarriage is really nature's safety measure for getting rid of a 'bad' pregnancy as early as possible. If some of the chromosomes are abnormal, or there are too few or too many of them, an abnormal message will result in an abnormal foetus being made. At least 38 per cent of early miscarriages when carefully studied show evidence of a chromosomal defect. The most common defects responsible are:

● *Three chromosomes of one type (instead of the normal pair)*. The defect is called 'trisomy' and the most frequently encountered trisomy is of chromosome number 16. This is usually due to a defective egg, and is therefore much more common in older women because they are more likely to ovulate eggs which are abnormal. When an early pregnancy is examined during an ultrasound scan, trisomy is classically associated with an empty sac (the membranes in which the baby should reside) or a very much smaller baby than expected.

Studies show that if a woman has had one miscarriage because of a trisomy, a second miscarriage is a bit more likely. If you have had a confirmed trisomic miscarriage, it might just be worth considering having amniocentesis or chorion villus sampling (see Chapter 14) in a subsequent pregnancy, because there is a slightly increased chance of an abnormal baby going to term.

● *One X-chromosome missing*. Normal girls have two X-chromosomes. Occasionally, one of the X-chromosomes may simply be missing (so-called 'monosomy'); this causes about 10–15 per cent of all miscarriages. Only about 1 per cent of pregnancies with one sex chromosome survive to birth. This defect in the few surviving children causes a condition called Turner's syndrome, which leads to deficient growth, absent periods and infertility.

● *Multiple or extra chromosomes*. This is also a common defect known as 'polyploidy'. The most common situation is where there is a complete extra set of chromosomes, which may be the result of an egg being fertilised by more than one sperm simultaneously. Many of these defects do not show in the baby in an early ultrasound scan, but there may be abnormalities of the placenta. Other babies show severe defects which are completely incompatible with life.

● *Changes in individual chromosomes*. These are a less common cause of miscarriage, occurring in less than 3 per cent. Some of these structural changes are inherited from one or other parent, who may carry a chromosomal abnormality even though they are perfectly 'normal' individuals. The defect can be in either partner. A blood test from both partners may be helpful in these rather rare cases.

Women who have miscarried may hear the term 'chromosomal translocation', which is one of the commoner structural changes in chromosomes. This occurs when part of one chromosome gets detached and reattaches to a different chromosome. The cause of this condition is unknown, but it is sometimes associated with exposure to radiation.

The commonest translocation associated with miscarriage is an exchange between a piece of chromosome 13 and chromosome 14. Such a translocation may be completely compatible with normal life, and many healthy adults have such a translocation. Unfortunately, translocations also may give rise to abnormal embryos, which sometimes miscarry. Screening of the blood white cells is usually needed to make a diagnosis and it is a matter of luck as to whether offspring may abort spontaneously. Although currently untreatable, there is hope that with embryo screening couples affected with this disorder may be able to have healthy pregnancies in future (*see* Chapter 14).

DIAGNOSING CHROMOSOMALLY DEFECTIVE MISCARRIAGES

Unfortunately chromosome studies have to be carried out on the aborted material to be sure that there was a genetic abnormality and this has to be done on very fresh tissue, which is frequently not available. Most miscarriages are not immediately shed from the womb, but 'stay put' for a few days after death has occurred. Moreover, these tests are quite unreliable if there is any trace of infection, and aborted material often contains bacteria. This is very frustrating for most couples, who dearly want to know what has caused their loss. Consequently, our knowledge about why someone has miscarried is frequently intuitive.

GENE DEFECTS

A few miscarriages may rarely be caused by a gene defect. Genes are the component part of each chromosome; there are several thousand on each chromosome. Some gene defects may cause miscarriage, but most result in the much more serious problem of an abnormal baby with a disease such as cystic fibrosis or muscular dystrophy.

HYDATIDIFORM MOLE

One odd cause of a miscarriage is a so-called 'hydatidiform mole'. This defect, caused by an abnormality of the chromosomes, causes a great deal of placental tissue to develop but with no foetus being formed. It is uncommon, occurring in about 1 in every 2,000 pregnancies in Britain. We know there is almost certainly an inherited tendency to produce molar pregnancy because in some communities – Malaysia, for example – it is much more common. It is also more frequent in older women.

Molar pregnancy often makes women feel very sick, because it produces very large amounts of the pregnancy hormone HCG. The uterus is generally quite a bit larger than would be expected by the length of the pregnancy; this is because the mole expands and dilates the uterus. Hydatidiform moles are actually tumours of the placental tissue, and the tissue produced looks like many little bunches of grapes; fortunately, this kind of tumour is very seldom malignant.

I suspect that some old stories of numerous multiple births were, in fact, aborted molar pregnancies. The most celebrated was that of Countess Margaret, daughter of Florent IV, the Earl of Holland, who gave birth on Good Friday in 1278 when she was forty-two years old (moles are commoner in older women). At that one birth, she delivered 365 infants – 182 boys, 182 girls and one hermaphrodite. They were all baptised in two large brazen dishes by the Bishop of Treras, all the boys being called John and the girls Elizabeth. Until the last century, the dishes were displayed in Losdun village church and were considered one of the great curiosities of Holland. Apparently (there is always a moral), the Countess had been stopped in a forest by a peasant woman carrying twins in her arms, asking for charity. The Countess rejected her haughtily, accusing her of having two babies by different fathers. The poor woman replied by cursing the Countess, praying that she have 'as many children as there are days in the year'.

Moles can very occasionally persist inside the uterus for several weeks or even months. The specialist may therefore want to conduct follow-up visits for some time after the event to make certain that the hormone HCG is no longer being made. It is very common for a small amount of residual molar tissue to take time to disappear, but usually no action is required. Sometimes people may be advised to avoid getting pregnant for several months after a molar pregnancy.

AGE

The age of the woman is an important factor in miscarriage. Apart from chromosome problems explained in Chapter 14, the older a woman is, the greater the proportion of abnormal eggs she will have in her ovaries. Such an egg can result in an embryo being formed which is not normal and not capable of becoming a proper pregnancy.

HORMONAL PROBLEMS

Miscarriage can occur if the right female hormones are not being produced in correct quantities or if a woman produces too much male hormone, testosterone. Some women who miscarry regularly do not make enough progesterone. This is the hormone which is made by the ovary in the *corpus luteum*, after ovulation, but it is also made by the placenta (afterbirth), by which the baby attaches itself to the uterus. Some doctors believe that a low blood progesterone level leads to miscarriage, but this is almost certainly untrue. If there is an abnormally low progesterone level in early pregnancy, this probably means the pregnancy is failing and not able to produce enough of this hormone. Consequently, giving extra progesterone, a very common treatment, is most unlikely to help.

Another hormonal problem that can cause miscarriage may occur if the blood level of luteinising hormone (LH, from the pituitary gland in the brain) is abnormally high or fluctuating. Abnormalities of LH can lead to the developing egg being matured abnormally, and this seems to lead to a miscarriage in some women. Abnormalities of LH hormone are common in women with polycystic ovaries. This is of very considerable interest and importance, because high levels of LH due to polycystic ovaries are now recognised to be a very common cause of miscarriage. Much of the credit for this observation must go to Dr Leslie Regan at St Mary's Hospital, London. She showed that high LH is associated with miscarriage, and because so many of these women do not ovulate very regularly, helped to explain why some women who are infertile sometimes also miscarry. Treatment is definitely possible if miscarriage is occurring because of high LH levels; these can be suppressed by taking the drug buserelin, following which ovulation can be induced with gonadotrophins (see p. 175).

There are, of course, other reasons why infertile women are prone to miscarriage, and these include abnormalities of the uterus (see below) and chromosomal abnormalities. Very rarely, other hormone problems such as thyroid abnormalities or diabetes may cause miscarriage. This is much less common than is often believed.

ABNORMALITIES OF THE UTERUS

These are an important and relatively common problem. If the uterus is misshapen, perhaps because of an abnormality from birth (this is surprisingly common), a developing pregnancy may end with a miscarriage. Sometimes benign swellings in the uterus, such as fibroids, may make its cavity irregular, and this also may prevent a pregnancy from implanting adequately.

Congenital abnormalities, such as a double uterus, are much more likely to cause miscarriage later in pregnancy, quite often after the twelfth week. They are also quite often associated with abnormalities of the cervix (when the cervix opens up prematurely – see below).

Adhesions inside the uterine cavity (see p. 110) may not only cause complete infertility but may also be associated with miscarriage.

CERVICAL INCOMPETENCE

The cervix, or neck of the uterus, is usually tightly closed, only opening a little to allow menstrual blood to escape and sperm to get in. Normally, during labour the cervix relaxes and opens wide to allow the baby in the womb to be born. However, some women have an open cervix ('cervical incompetence' is its medical name). This may be an inborn fault, the result of surgical injury, or follows a previous pregnancy. The muscles of the cervix may be weak, opening the cervical canal to let bacteria in. The infection can then inflame the membranes surrounding the baby and a miscarriage usually results.

Miscarriages caused by an open cervix usually occur quite late in pregnancy, after the fourteenth week and, more usually, after the sixteenth week.

INTRAUTERINE DEVICE (IUD, 'COIL') IN PLACE

It is actually possible very occasionally to get pregnant with a coil in place – a rare but sometimes distressing occurrence – with a slightly increased risk of miscarrying. Having said that, most pregnancies in this situation continue to term and there is no evidence at all that any baby will be abnormal because it shared the uterus with a coil. Stories about babies being delivered waving a coil in their fist are probably apocryphal. Usually any retained coil is delivered with the placenta.

ENVIRONMENTAL HAZARDS

It is widely thought that various chemicals may cause miscarriage. One notorious example is Dioxin – recalled the dreadful chemical factory accident in Italy which resulted in many woman subsequently miscarrying their pregnancies. Wheat contaminated with lead, regrettably sent by a famine relief organisation, caused some women to miscarry in Africa in the early 1980s. Some insecticides are dangerous, and intimate contact with other severe poisons in early pregnancy is probably undesirable. Certain drugs are also dangerous. The classic example is Thalidomide, the sleeping pill, which caused many miscarriages and the birth of children with defective limbs.

Radiation is harmful during early pregnancy. Both Hiroshima and the recent nuclear accident in the USSR at Chernobyl resulted in some women miscarrying early pregnancies. There is no evidence, however, that using a microwave oven, computer screen or wordprocessor in early pregnancy is harmful.

Smoking in early pregnancy is stupid if one is prone to miscarriages. There is also good evidence that marijuana (cannabis) usage can lead to loss of a pregnancy. Heavy drinking of alcohol may also cause miscarriage; chronic alcoholics tend to have more miscarriages and more abnormal children.

INFECTIONS

Several different bacteria and some viruses are thought to be responsible for very occasional miscarriages in both humans and animals. None of these germs regularly causes a problem, and exactly how rarely or commonly they cause pregnancy loss is uncertain. The most important viral infection is German measles (Rubella), and young women who have not had this mild disease are well advised to get immunised against it, so that they have no risk on getting pregnant. The doctor will certainly screen for infection if this is indicated.

ACUTE AND CHRONIC ILLNESS

Very occasionally, an acute illness may cause miscarriage, usually because a high fever has damaged an early developing pregnancy. Most common is probably severe influenza. Chronic illnesses which may rarely cause miscarriage are high blood pressure, severe kidney disease and some rare auto-immune diseases such as lupus. With all these diseases, normal pregnancy is more usual so there is no need for great worry.

IMMUNOLOGICAL PROBLEMS

There are three ways in which immune problems might cause miscarriage:

1.   First, there is some evidence that some women miscarry if they share similar tissue types to their partner. The developing baby is immunologically very curious. All its tissues are unique

to it alone; it is quite different from its mother and yet, in spite of contact with the mother's blood supply, it is not rejected. Any other foreign tissue – for example, a kidney, skin, even bacteria – would be immediately rejected by any human with an intact immune system. It is a considerable mystery why a baby is not treated by its mother's body in the same way. For years, it was thought that the womb might be immunologically 'privileged' and that foreign things in it would not be rejected; this is now clearly untrue. Some researchers have supposed that pregnancy itself might change a mother's rejection response, but this is certainly not the whole story because tissues grafted on to pregnant women are rejected in the same way as they would be in non-pregnant individuals.

For some time, it has been thought that certain miscarriages may be caused by problems in the immune system – that is, miscarriage results from a kind of rejection response in the body of the mother. Curiously, this rejection seems more likely if mother and father have similar tissue types. Evidence in animals shows that inbreeding between close relatives can produce a much higher rate of early pregnancy loss.

If there is a degree of compatibility between male and female partners, a few doctors recommend a form of immunisation of the mother if she is prone to regular miscarriage. A transfusion of cells from the father is given to his partner in a relatively simple treatment. I must emphasise that I personally am extremely dubious about the value of this treatment. Moreover, I have seen some women who seem to have become sterile after this treatment; before treatment, they miscarried regularly, but after treatment, they could not conceive at all. What is clear is that there are no really good figures which prove the value of this immune therapy. I am also particularly sceptical because none of the few 'eminent' doctors dishing out this therapy can explain why it should work or the precise statistical basis for their results. The history of immune therapy is full of magic cures, few of which have stood the test of time.

2. Very rarely a miscarriage may occur if there is severe incompatibility of blood groups between mother and father. The classic example is severe Rhesus disease, which nowadays

is very uncommon in this country indeed. A simple blood test can be done to see if this is the cause.

3. One type of immune defect which has now been incriminated in miscarriage is the presence of certain tissue antibodies, in particular so-called lupus anticoagulant or anti-cardiolipin antibodies. It seems that the presence of these antibodies means that the blood vessels of the placenta may be attacked and abortion can, on occasion, occur relatively late in pregnancy, sometimes even after the twentieth week. A relatively simple blood test can be done which is helpful in finding the cause. Various treatments have been tried, and it is thought that aspirin tablets, and possibly injections of heparin which prevent blood from clotting, may be beneficial. It is important to understand that patients with these conditions can go on to have healthy pregnancies but that this treatment may also help.

ABNORMAL BLOOD SUPPLY OR CHEMISTRY IN THE UTERUS

There is growing evidence that an abnormal blood supply in the uterus, or deficiencies in its chemistry, may be quite important as the cause of some miscarriages. Scientific work in this area is very new, but there are likely to be important developments in this area within the next few years.

STRESS AND PSYCHOLOGICAL FACTORS

This is very difficult to evaluate, but is important because the cause of so many miscarriages is unclear. However, women who are prone to miscarry have less risk of miscarrying again if they are looked after with tenderness and care in a subsequent pregnancy. The precise therapy that a woman receives may not actually matter; it is most interesting that simple reassurance (irrespective of any well-defined treatments) may be particularly therapeutic.

PREVENTING A MISCARRIAGE:
GENERAL MEASURES

REST

The more one relaxes and takes it easy, the better the blood flow to the baby and the more quiet the uterus will be. It is best to get up late and retire early. Perhaps time off work will be sensible, at least until the pregnancy is firmly established, at about ten weeks or so. People who repeatedly miscarry at a particular time should aim to take it really easy at that stage. Women in this situation should not think of themselves as invalids though; refusing to leave the house and avoiding any social life at all may make one more tense and are not likely to help.

Doctors sometimes may suggest a period of rest in hospital, particularly when a woman in early pregnancy has had several repeated miscarriages. Although hospitals are hardly ever relaxing places, hospital bedrest is an option that is worth a try. Figures show that this is one of the best ways of helping women who have had several miscarriages.

AVOIDING CONSTIPATION

It is faintly possible that straining very heavily to pass a constipated motion might just endanger a pregnancy which is already at risk of miscarriage. For this reason, some doctors advise extra fibre in the diet (such as wholemeal bread, fruit and vegetables), and they may also suggest a little senna to keep the bowel regular. A doctor can give advice about which laxatives are safe.

IRON AND FOLIC ACID TABLETS

Although people say that being short of iron makes miscarriage more likely, this is generally untrue. If a pregnant woman is not anaemic, iron supplements are quite unnecessary until about the twenty-eighth week.

Some clinics prescribe a small amount of folic acid. This causes no upset and is the one vitamin that may be genuinely valuable.

ALCOHOL AND SMOKING

A little alcohol (one or two drinks a week) is not harmful and may even help by increasing relaxation, and by quietening the uterus. Smoking may reduce the blood supply to the baby.

TRAVEL

It is best to avoid travel in early pregnancy, if one is prone to miscarriage. Short, untiring journeys are fine, and gentle train journeys will do no harm. However, it is really foolish to go on long flights or skiing holidays in early pregnancy if there is any threat of miscarriage.

MAKING LOVE

People who have regularly miscarried probably should avoid sex in the early pregnancy, at least until about the twelfth to fourteenth week. One should not spend the rest of the week feeling guilty if one suddenly feels very amorous and gets carried away. The chances of miscarriage are very remote.

SPORT

This is best avoided. A little gentle swimming will do no harm but avoid tennis or more strenuous sports.

Many women blame themselves for miscarrying. They feel that if only they had done less, rested more or altered their lives in some way, the loss could have been avoided. This is wrong. Although I have suggested various ways of self-help, it can't be denied that the effect of all these measures is marginal. The truth is that it is very hard to damage a normal pregnancy, no matter what one does.

PREVENTING MISCARRIAGE: SPECIAL TREATMENT

GENETIC CAUSES

Tests can be done on the miscarried embryo to see if the chromosomes are normal. Parents can also be screened by blood tests. If the blood tests are abnormal, the clinic will give advice about the likelihood of repeated miscarriage.

HORMONAL PROBLEMS

If there is a hormonal imbalance, it too can be detected by blood tests before pregnancy and corrected with hormone treatment.

Progesterone is sometimes prescribed after ovulation, either in the form of an injection or pessaries (which one can put into the vagina at night). The treatment is controversial because many experts think that 'replacement' therapy of this sort is neither effective nor necessary.

UTERINE ABNORMALITIES

These can easily be detected by X-rays (hysterosalpingograms) and then treated surgically (*see* Chapter 8).

CERVICAL INCOMPETENCE

This can be treated by a repair of the cervix before getting pregnant, or by it being stitched shut afterwards. Most doctors much prefer the latter. Although this may seem like shutting the stable door a bit too late, it is the safer and more effective treatment. Stitches are put in at around fourteen weeks, before cervical incompetence can cause miscarriage, and must be removed before giving birth; this does not require anaesthesia.

IMMUNE PROBLEMS

There is increasing evidence that regular, daily doses of aspirin may be quite effective in early pregnancy to prevent miscarriage. This is a simple treatment, which may work by changing the clotting which can occur in placental tissues. We are impressed with this approach.

COPING WITH MISCARRIAGE

Having a miscarriage at any time is a severe shock.

If you are a woman in this situation, you naturally feel a loss of life within you, as well as an event which makes you unwell and depressed. This is much worse if you have had difficulty getting pregnant or if you have already had a miscarriage. Doctors and friends feel helpless and are only able to offer platitudes. Because doctors are trained to heal people, they find it very difficult to deal with this condition, which occurs so often in spite of treatment, and perhaps after weeks of rest, and, when it does, is so frequently inexplicable. This makes mere words sound pointless. Friends often offer clichés: 'At least you didn't know the baby' or 'Lucky that you've got other children'. One infertile patient of mine was told by her best friend: 'Don't think about it and it'll soon be all over.' Such advice, though common, is remarkably unhelpful.

To make matters worse, what happens when a miscarriage occurs can be a cause for unhappiness. Apart from childbirth, miscarriage is about the most common reason for a younger woman to enter hospital. For this very reason hospital staff unfortunately tend to treat miscarriage as routine and do not always seem as helpful as they might be. For one thing, many doctors and nurses cannot quite understand why you may feel so frightened. Very often they are perfectly kind and reassuring but don't seem to understand that you have lost a baby that was very real to you. Because the vast majority of women who miscarry go on to have a perfectly normal pregnancy within a few months, hospital staff sometimes appear a little unaware of their distress.

Having a miscarriage frequently means staying in hospital and possibly having an anaesthetic so that the remnants of the pregnancy can be removed. Frequently in the past, women who were miscarrying were admitted to obstetric units where other women were expecting a happy outcome to their pregnancies. Fortunately, things nowadays are rather better organised, even if we, as a profession, are slow to accept the severity of the trauma involved in miscarrying.

Many difficult emotions come to a head with a miscarriage. It is absolutely usual to ask yourself if you were to blame. It is rare not to be able to think of innumerable things that you might have done to yourself, which have resulted in losing your baby. This feeling is very seldom justified. Women commonly believe that sexual activity, staying at work, stress, a sudden fall or smoking a cigarette may have brought on the miscarriage. While this kind of thinking is natural, it is very rare for any of these factors to be of any importance.

Apart from feelings of sadness and guilt, anger is a common emotion. However, there is little rational basis for this – it is seldom indeed that anybody can be said to have caused a miscarriage. Nevertheless, it is worth knowing that your unreasonable feelings of anger are a natural reaction to what seems to be an unnatural event.

I think it is essential to recognise that a miscarriage is a loss of life and not something that can be brushed away. You have been bereaved, and it is important to cry, to mourn. Some women find it helpful to see the placenta or remnants of their conception. Seeing the tissue, or the embryo, helps many come to terms with their loss. Hospital staff may be a little wary of this, but you or your partner may ask to see if this is possible.

Grieving in itself is the most important part of the healing process. You both will naturally feel particularly anxious and nervous during a future pregnancy, but there are some very positive things to be remembered. The figures clearly show that even women who miscarry many, many times are likely eventu-

278 PROBLEMS DURING EARLY PREGNANCY

ally to conceive normally. You may need to ask yourself how far you are prepared to try, how much trauma you are able to take. I have seen several women have normal deliveries after ten or twelve miscarriages.[38] Of course, if you do persist and succeed eventually, this will not wipe out your earlier distress, but it will not have been in vain.

TELLING YOUR CHILDREN

Very often you will have the difficult problem of telling your children that you have lost an early pregnancy. Listen carefully to what they say and ask questions to find out what they are thinking. Show them affection, while explaining gently in a simple, direct manner what has happened to the baby; don't necessarily avoid using words like 'death' or 'died'. There is no reason not to say why you are sad, but avoid showing that you are frightened or anxious. You must also recognise that your children may well not want to talk about things immediately, but that their questions may surface later. At all times, reassure your children that they are not the cause of what happened, and are in no danger at all. The fact that you have been away in hospital may mean that your children feel that being abandoned is a possibility in future. Many children may show quite strong signs of emotional disturbance, especially sleeplessness, anger, bed-wetting, nightmares, sudden fright or anxiety, and you should be ready to be very supportive.

[38] I am reminded of a delightful Hungarian lady whom I looked after as a young house-surgeon under the late Professor John McClure Browne's instruction. Following a damaging termination of pregnancy in Budapest (where the state used to encourage abortion as a form of contraception), she had fifteen miscarriages. I thought my boss was fairly stupid in persisting in admitting her to hospital in each early pregnancy. He simply said that she would eventually have a normal pregnancy if we continued to admit her. I actually was brash enough to argue with him until her sixteenth pregnancy when, after prolonged bedrest, she delivered a little girl at the age of forty-two.

THE MAN

Men, too, have a very difficult time when their partner miscarries. The majority worry most about the woman's safety: 'What if she bleeds to death?' is a common but unspoken question. Men also feel sad or disappointed. Very often their grief will not be as acute, and they may find it difficult to understand why their partner feels so deeply. Many men also feel angry: 'Why us?' is commonly asked. Others resent the need for them to be the strong or supportive partner: 'I'm feeling the pain as well.' Disbelief is a very common feeling, as is a general sensation of pessimism – 'Will we ever have a baby?' – especially if there was difficulty in conceiving in the first place. Feelings of guilt are also frequent in men. Sometimes this may be guilt at not feeling very distressed, or even being relieved at the loss of the pregnancy. At other times, the guilt may be because he feels that he may have caused the miscarriage by making love or by not taking sufficient care of his partner in other ways. Men also need to grieve and cry, but many feel quite inhibited about this and, curiously, the female partner may have to be quite supportive in this situation.

IS THERE ANY HOPE?

If you have been infertile as a result of tubal disease or a hormonal problem, a miscarriage is proof that you can get pregnant. As a result, you should see this as a sign of real hope that you can conceive. We have analysed the figures for women who miscarry after tubal surgery or in vitro fertilisation, and it is clear that, provided treatment is continued, the chances of a successful pregnancy are much better than 50: 50. Remember that a miscarriage is sure evidence that your tubes are open, that you do ovulate and that your partner's sperm are fertile.

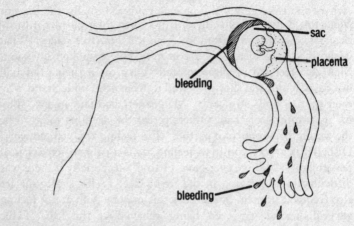

An ectopic pregnancy in the right tube.

TRYING TO UNDERSTAND WHY IT HAPPENED

It is natural to feel confused after a miscarriage, and, if you are in this situation, it may take some time before you really are ready to think of why it occurred. One of the problems is that, most of the time, the precise reason for a particular miscarriage is unknown. Hopefully, the bewildering list of causes I have given earlier will help people to ask the right questions and, if necessary, seek investigation to reduce the risk of it happening again.

Ectopic Pregnancy

An ectopic pregnancy is a pregnancy outside the uterine cavity. After fertilisation, the egg does not manage to travel as far as the uterus, but stops on the way and it sticks and grows there. The usual place is the Fallopian tube (about 96 per cent), but occasionally implantation happens in other places – the ovary, abdominal cavity outside the uterus or the wall of the uterus where the tube enters the uterine cavity. Usually the placenta (afterbirth) cannot form normally. As a result, virtually all ectopic pregnancies die, or they start to bleed vigorously. This is very similar to a miscarriage, except that the bleeding is internal and occasionally can be so heavy that the situation becomes life-threatening.

Ectopic pregnancies are common; in the United Kingdom, at least 1 in 200 pregnancies implants outside the uterus. The incidence of ectopic pregnancies may be rising, possibly because many women have damaged Fallopian tubes which predispose to this problem.

Although having an ectopic pregnancy is an extremely upsetting event – even worse than having a miscarriage because of the pain and shock – it is worth remembering that women who have ectopics have demonstrated an ability to get pregnant. Like a miscarriage, this shows that they are ovulating, that their partner's sperm is fertile and that the eggs are capable of forming embryos. We find it most worth while to treat women who have previously had ectopics, as often the outlook for a successful pregnancy in the end is often better than for other infertile women.

WHAT ARE THE SYMPTOMS?

Usually there is quite a lot of pain, often to one side of the abdomen, together with light bleeding from the vagina. Quite frequently the pain is 'crampy' – that is, it comes in waves. The pain generally starts before there is any bleeding. Most women feel pregnant and normally a pregnancy test will be positive, unless the pregnancy has already started to die. If there is any internal bleeding, this can cause one to feel unwell – possibly sick and giddy or faint.

All these symptoms are likely to occur early in pregnancy; indeed an ectopic pregnancy can occur even when there has not been a missed period. It is rare after the tenth week, so if any of the symptoms I have described occur later in pregnancy, they probably indicate a miscarriage. It is vital to contact the doctor if there are any of these symptoms.

Very often the diagnosis of ectopic pregnancy depends on the previous medical history (*see* below).

WHAT CAUSES AN ECTOPIC PREGNANCY?

This is not fully understood. These conditions make it more likely:

● If the tube is damaged by previous infection, or is partly blocked, an ectopic pregnancy can implant in a scarred part of the tube. This is the most common reason for an ectopic and accounts for probably 95 per cent of ectopic pregnancies.

● After embryos have been placed in the uterus during IVF, one of them may leave the uterus spontaneously and move into a tube, where it may implant. This is much more likely if the tubes are already damaged. Although people often believe that IVF is a way of avoiding the risk of an ectopic pregnancy, the incidence of ectopic pregnancy after IVF in women with damaged tubes is just as high as it is after tubal surgery.

● Some women who have worn an intrauterine device – an IUD or 'coil' – are prone to ectopic pregnancy. This may be because the coil causes some low-grade infection, leading perhaps to damage of the lining of the tube.

● Women who have already had one ectopic pregnancy are rather more likely to have another, because one of the tubes is invariably damaged.

DIAGNOSIS AND TREATMENT OF
ECTOPIC PREGNANCY

The diagnosis of ectopic pregnancy can be difficult, although it has been made much easier in recent years because of various tests that are now available. The doctor will want to do a special pregnancy test (probably a blood test) to detect very small amounts of the pregnancy hormone HCG. Ultrasound scans can be very helpful. Nowadays vaginal ultrasound is frequently used because it gives a very accurate idea of whether there is any swelling in one or other tube. If there is any doubt about the diagnosis, laparoscopy remains the most important investigation for ectopic pregnancy.

It is not wise to leave an ectopic pregnancy inside the body once a diagnosis has been firmly made; for one thing, it can virtually never grow to a viable size. An operation is needed to remove it. Most units like to perform a laparoscopy first, and then, if an ectopic pregnancy is present, an operation is carried out to remove it.

One of the difficulties about the surgery is that the ectopic pregnancy may have damaged the tube very considerably, even if it was previously normal. As a result, surgeons often prefer to remove both the embryo and the tube it is in, particularly if that tube is rather badly damaged. While this means that another ectopic cannot implant in that tube it also means there now is only one tube to get pregnant with in future. Therefore, some surgeons try to remove the embryo alone and preserve the tube. This 'conservative' surgery is done increasingly frequently nowadays if the woman is already infertile or if there is trouble with the other tube which may increase the chance of infertility. Although preserving the tube increases the possibility of another ectopic pregnancy (thanks to modern techniques, the risk does not seem to be that greatly increased), it does give a better chance of normal pregnancy as well.

Removal of ectopic pregnancy usually requires an open operation which leaves a cut in the abdomen, rather similar to that used for tubal microsurgery (see p. 178). Because ectopic pregnancies sometimes bleed quite vigorously, blood transfusion may be recommended. The operation is obviously relatively major, and it will take time to recover from it. It is quite like having the appendix removed and is not dangerous, but it means staying in hospital for about a week.

LAPAROSCOPIC REMOVAL

Some centres in Britain, the United States and France remove ectopic pregnancies without opening the abdomen; instead, the pregnancy is sucked out of the affected tube during a laparoscopic examination. This technique is suitable if the pregnancy is quite early (and therefore small). I am very impressed with this approach, as it involves less surgery and trauma. Unfortunately, most hospitals in the UK are, at present, unable to perform the laparoscopic removal of ectopic pregnancies. A doctor will advise this approach only if he or she has the special expertise required and has access to the right instruments.

INJECTION OF METHOTREXATE

Another approach to treating ectopic pregnancy which avoids major surgery is the injection of drugs into the ectopic pregnancy itself which stop it growing and cause it to perish. The drug which is most widely used is methotrexate, which specifically stops the placental tissues from developing. At Hammersmith we favour this approach when possible, because it causes much less disturbance to women. Usually the injection is done using a laparoscope, under general anaesthetic. Alternatively, some units have done these injections simply using the ultrasound machine to guide them; this has the advantage that general anaesthesia is not needed. After the injection the patient is rested in bed for a day or so, and then may be allowed home once there is confirmation that the ectopic is no longer growing. We have now had the opportunity to examine the tubes of a number of women who had a methotrexate injection, many months after the treatment for an ectopic. Healing seems excellent, which is very encouraging.

At present, it is not possible to take an ectopic pregnancy out of a tube and immediately replace it in the uterus. The problem is that, although the embryo may be normal, its blood supply would not regrow.

COPING WITH AN ECTOPIC PREGNANCY

Having an ectopic pregnancy is a severely traumatic experience. Many of the problems that are raised are similar to those caused by miscarriage. However, an ectopic pregnancy means a surgical procedure, which adds greatly to the upset. Unfortunately, the severity of a woman's distress is not always fully appreciated by medical and nursing staff. Because ectopic pregnancy is still largely a surgical 'emergency', doctors tend to focus on the need to 'save the patient's life'. This anxiety is invariably communicated to relatives and friends, compounding the problem. The fact that a baby has been lost is often forgotten. Far too often, doctors are happy to say 'we saved her life', neglecting the loss to the woman.

In fact, the risk involved in having an ectopic pregnancy is pretty negligible nowadays, though many patients prone to this complication live in fear of it. Modern diagnostic methods, especially laparoscopy and ultrasound, mean that ectopic pregnancy can be diagnosed very early and that the risk of significant haemorrhage is really very small. Except in rare cases where a Fallopian tube containing an ectopic pregnancy ruptures, causing life-threatening internal bleeding, removal of an ectopic pregnancy is certainly no more (and probably less) dangerous than having an appendix removed.

Because early diagnosis is now more common, the death of a pregnancy may be even more remote in the mind of a doctor or nurse. Early diagnosis means that damage is limited and surgery may often save the tube. While it may be reassuring to the woman to know that her tube is preserved, emphasis may shift away from the fact that a much-wanted baby has died.

WHAT ARE THE CHANCES OF HAVING A SECOND ECTOPIC PREGNANCY?

Women who have already had one ectopic pregnancy are about ten times more likely to have another. Even so, the odds are about 25 to 1 against, so a normal pregnancy is still much more likely than a second ectopic. It is important to remember this, because mamy women become so worried about the risk of another tubal pregnancy that they use contraception indefinitely. Normal pregnancy is quite possible even after several ectopics.

> Eleni, a thirty-year-old patient of mine, had had one ectopic pregnancy and her right tube had been partly removed during the operation to remove the embryo. I did some tubal surgery to repair her right tube as far as I could. She subsequently had two more ectopics, one in each tube, spaced nine months apart. Nothing daunted, she came back to see me, insisting on further tubal surgery. I told her that she was a very brave woman, but that there was no point in yet another abdominal operation. However, she eventually persuaded me to 'have a go'. During microsurgery I was able to repair her left tube to some extent. Since the operation she has had three babies, all girls, now aged eight, five and three. I have no idea which of her appalling-looking tubes managed to transport the embryos into the uterus.

Sometimes women find that they are unable to conceive again after an ectopic pregnancy. If this is the problem, the best thing is to have laparoscopy done to check the tubes. An ectopic often results in some adhesions forming, and it is a simple matter to check on this; it may even be possible to have the problem sorted out at the same time, with the adhesions being cut during laparoscopy. Alternatively, it may be possible to repair the other tube with only a tiny risk of another ectopic. A third possibility will be IVF treatment (see Chapter 11), which has a comparatively high success rate after ectopic pregnancy.

CHAPTER FOURTEEN

Coping with Genetic Diseases

The greatest worry that all pregnant women have is 'Will my baby be normal?' We are now increasingly able to detect and prevent genetic diseases before and during pregnancy, and there has been a number of exciting developments which help ensure the health of babies.

It is probably no exaggeration to say that genetic disease is now the single greatest unsolved problem of modern medicine. A child born with a genetic disease will have that problem for life. Of course, a few birth defects may be surgically correctable, but when the body's chemistry is involved even surgery is unlikely to help. Many of these diseases, if not most, give rise to distressing chronic physical and mental handicap, and they are the second most common cause of babies dying at birth. In spite of the availability of screening, 1 in 50 babies are born in Britain with a major genetic defect, a typical example being spina bifida. About 1 in 100 babies have a serious or defective gene. Most of these gene defects are inherited, but a few may occur out of the blue when there is no family background or history suggesting a particular disease. These 'bolts of lightning' are so-called 'gene mutations'. Occasionally, in about 1 in 200 babies, there may be a problem with a whole chromosome (or part of one), which carries many genes. Such a disease is Down's syndrome.

If these gruesome statistics were not enough, it is worth considering that about 25 per cent of all children occupying a hospital bed are there because of a genetic problem. As a result, genetic disease puts a great burden on health services, as well as upon the social and educational services. Moreover, they cause difficulties and much misery for the families of affected children.

The problem of genetic disease goes further than just in children. A recent study in Britain showed that, in one average large general hospital, no less than 12 per cent of all adult in-patients were there because of a disease which was genetically related. Some genetic diseases do not surface until adulthood; others may not appear until then if they are not severe. In addition, many of the major health problems facing society have at least a genetic component – diabetes, cancer, heart attacks and much mental illness all have important contributing genetic factors.

What exactly is genetic disease?

There are two rather confusing terms. First, there is 'congenital malformation'. This is a defect with which a baby is born; it is occasionally, but by no mean always, inherited. Second, there is 'genetic defect'. This is an inherited defect resulting from the action of genes.

In Chapter 1, I described the twenty-three pairs of chromosomes in each cell of the body. One of each pair of chromosomes is inherited randomly from each parent. Each chromosome carries thousands of genes, each one of which is a code for a specific characteristic. Some of the characteristics produced by genes are trivial – for example, there is a gene which can give rise to blue eyes – but most others are much more important because they control basic functions of the body.

Genes, which are assembled in pairs along each chromosome, are said to be *dominant* or *recessive*. If in a pair of genes one or both are dominant and present, this produces a recognisable effect in the body. As for recessive genes, they only produce a notice-able effect if *both* of the pair are present. Most diseases inherited via genes are carried by recessive genes. Such recessive genes are often common, but individuals will be born with a particular disease associated with a recessive gene only if both their parents carried that particular gene and both passed it on to their child. An exception to this general rule is if an individual is born with a mutant gene, arising anew as a result of fresh chemical action. He or she may be affected with a particular genetic disease, even though the parents were not genetic carriers.

A genetic disorder can be one of four different types:

SINGLE GENE DEFECTS

The number of diseases caused by single defective genes is, curiously, not precisely known, although it is estimated that there are about 4,000. Roughly half of these are caused by dominant genes, rather fewer by recessive genes and the remainder are sex-linked – that is, they are carried on the X-chromosome and their inheritance depends on the sex of the baby.

DOMINANT GENETIC DISEASE

Most diseases caused by dominant genes are rare. This is because, if the gene is present, the offspring will have the disease and die before being able to reproduce. The exceptions are if the dominant gene does not produce a fatal disease, or if the disease is not severe enough to prevent a sexual relationship or pregnancy. The most common dominant genetic disease is probably hypercholesterolaemia, an abnormally high level of cholesterol in the blood which leads to early death in young adults (in their twenties and onwards) from heart attacks. This occurs in 1 in 500 births. Another well-known disease is Huntington's chorea, occurring in 1 in 2,000 births, causing loss of muscle control, dementia and death in middle age. This is a terrifying disease to have in the family, because members of the family, who have intimate knowledge of its appalling consequences, have to wait to find out whether they also have this dominant gene. If they do, they will start to experience themselves the horrifying deterioration that they have previously witnessed in a loved one.

RECESSIVE GENETIC DISEASE

The most common recessive genetic disease is cystic fibrosis, carried by 1 in 20 of the population. Because both parents need to have a recessive gene for their children to have the actual disease, 1 in 400 couples (20 × 20) are at risk of having a child with this illness. Cystic fibrosis causes deficient digestion and recurrent chest infections. This does not sound so bad, but the disease usually requires multiple hospital admissions and daily treatments, and the majority of sufferers die in childhood, though some survive (usually very disabled) into young adult life. Apart from the hardship to the sufferers and their families, it has been estimated that it costs up to £15,000 annually to keep a child with this illness alive.

Some recessive genetic diseases are much more common in certain parts of the world or in certain racial (and interrelated) groups. Thalassaemia, a very serious blood disease causing severe disability, is a typical example. Although it only occurs in 1 in 20,000 births in the general population, it is very common in people of Mediterranean origin. For example, 1 in 50 babies born to Cypriots living in London suffers from this terrible illness. At least 200,000 babies are born annually around the world with this disease; in Thailand alone there are thought to be some 500,000 children suffering from some form of thalassaemia. Most of these, in spite of inadequate but expensive treatment, will die by the age of five.

SEX-LINKED DISEASE

The sex-linked diseases are usually passed on by females but only boys are affected. The most important of these is Duchenne muscular dystrophy, which causes progressive muscular weakness. One in 5,000 boys born in Britain suffers from it. These children are usually confined to wheelchairs; death occurs when they can no longer use their breathing muscles. A disease that is better known (though less common) is haemophilia, which has attracted popular attention because this was the notorious disease that afflicted the unfortunate Russian royal family and was carried by Queen Victoria. The blood of haemophiliacs does not clot properly, and they are therefore in danger of uncontrolled bleeding. This can be avoided if they take Factor VIII, a component of blood.

Chromosome defects

Chromosomes are paired. Each of the twenty-three chromosome pairs is classified according to size, chromosome pair no. 1 being the biggest and pair no. 22 the smallest. Pair no. 23 is composed of the sex chromosomes, XX or XY. Diseases caused by chromosome defects occur when one or more chromosomes carrying many genes are abnormal. Instead of a normal pair of chromosomes there may be three; alternatively, one of a pair may be missing (*see* Turner's syndrome, p. 103). Occasionally only a piece of a chromosome may be missing. Sometimes, one chromosome from one pair may be mixed with that of another.

Most chromosome abnormalities, because they involve several and not just one gene defect, are incompatible with life. Consequently, most pregnancies with a chromosome defect end with a miscarriage – nature's 'safety valve'. It seems extraordinary that, overall, 15 per cent of all pregnancies that end in a birth involve a chromosome defect, that is about 1 in 190 babies. When you consider how common chromosome defects are, it is astonishing how little we know about the causes. We know that abnormal eggs, especially in older women, are likely to result in an embryo with three copies of chromosome 21 which results in Down's syndrome (*see* p. 87). Although it is thought that radiation, some chemicals and a few other environmental factors may cause some chromosome defects, the cause of most is entirely unclear. This remains a major area for research.

Congenital malformations

Some congenital malformations have a genetic origin. When they do, it is usually because several 'bad' genes are acting together. Consequently, their inheritance does not follow any precise pattern, but people who have given birth to a baby with certain genetic defects may have a high chance of conceiving another affected child – probably a risk of about 1 in 20. An example of a very common disease with a strong genetic component is spina bifida, a 'neural tube defect' in which part of the spinal cord bulges out of a gap in the backbone. Children with this disorder may, if they survive, be confined to a wheelchair and have defective bladder and bowel function.

Not all congenital malformations are genetic. Some are due to viruses. Others may be due to exposure to radiation, vitamin deficiency, chemicals or drugs. An example of the latter is, of course, Thalidomide. It is most important to recognise that most malformations occur as a matter of pure chance. Far too frequently, people blame themselves for what has happened to their children.

Illnesses with a genetic component

These illnesses are indeed numerous. Diabetes, which occurs in about half of one per cent of the population, is one. Schizophrenia, affecting 1 per cent, is another. The list is extensive, and includes coronary heart disease, arthritis, multiple sclerosis, certain types of infertility (especially those associated with defects of the ovary or uterus), some forms of mental retardation, and some of the rarer types of cancer. All these illnesses are probably caused, at least in part, by several genes acting together in the body.

Preventing genetic disease

Only a minority of genetic diseases can be effectively treated. Prevention remains the biggest weapon we have in fighting genetic diseases. It can be accomplished in two ways. Using modern methods of chemical or DNA analysis (DNA being the material from which chromosomes are made), couples can be screened before conceiving and then counselled. Unfortunately, this type of screening is presently only possible for very few diseases. Moreover, because these diseases usually arise from two parents with the same recessive gene, the best prevention that can be achieved is by advising such couples not to have children. The other method of prevention involves identifying couples at risk, and offering to terminate any pregnancy which may be affected.

Neither of these is satisfactory. Genetic counselling is limited because there are few diseases we can identify in prospective parents. On the other hand, termination of pregnancy is fraught with ethical and emotional problems. Apart from any moral arguments against killing a foetus, so-called 'therapeutic abortion' is also harsh for the mother. The effect that terminating a pregnancy has on women (and indeed men) has tended to be trivialised by our society. Apart from medical complications, which are not that infrequent, nearly all women feel very sad and are often profoundly depressed following termination. These feelings can be much deeper than is often supposed and some couples feel permanent grief at the deliberate termination of a pregnancy. Apart from any religious considerations, this, I believe, is why there has been a growing realisation that bringing up a handicapped child may be preferable for some couples.

Antenatal diagnosis

AMNIOCENTESIS

Many genetic defects can be diagnosed in time to consider termination of the pregnancy and amniocentesis is the most common diagnostic method. It involves taking some fluid from the sac surrounding the baby. The cells from the baby can be analysed as well as any chemicals it excretes.

Most chromosomal defects can be identified reasonably reliably by this method. Many other defects which involve abnormal body chemistry can also be detected, provided, of course, that the doctors know for which chemicals to test; an example is Tay-Sachs disease (which causes babies to die from progressive brain deterioration by the age of two years). Amniocentesis is a very safe procedure in good hands, carrying only perhaps a 1 in 200 chance of starting a miscarriage.

The disadvantages of amniocentesis are that the sac surrounding the baby is not usually big enough for safe sampling until about the fourteenth or sixteenth week of pregnancy. Moreover, because there are only very few cells floating in the amniotic fluid, they have to be grown in a culture before a chromosome test can be done reliably; this may take three weeks or more. If there is a chromosomal defect, the pregnancy may be very advanced, perhaps nineteen weeks at the earliest before a decision to terminate can be made. This can be very traumatic because, by this time, the baby can be felt moving and there is inevitably a commitment to being pregnant. Moreover, termination involves going through a form of labour, which is obviously very unpleasant.

CHORION VILLUS SAMPLING

Recently, another method for antenatal diagnosis has been developed. Chorion villus sampling – called CVS for short –

involves taking a small piece from the baby's side of the placenta away for analysis. Because both the baby and its placental tissue derive from the same cells, cells from the placenta accurately reflect the condition of the baby. CVS can be done either by sucking a few placental cells away through a tube inserted through the cervix, or by inserting a needle through the woman's abdominal wall. With the latter technique (and sometimes the former), ultrasound is used to guide the doctor so that the baby and its membranes are left undamaged.

CVS can be done much earlier in pregnancy than amniocentesis, usually between eight and eleven weeks. Moreover, diagnosis of many defects is fairly rapid, particularly when a specific gene defect is suspected. Modern methods of DNA analysis mean that a diagnosis should not take longer than two weeks; indeed, much more rapid methods are now available. Using a new method called *polymerase chain reaction* (PCR), many gene defects can be diagnosed within twenty-four hours. The advantages are considerable, because termination of an early pregnancy is much less traumatic. Also, if PCR can be used, the emotional stress of waiting for a diagnosis is substantially reduced. CVS can also be used for testing for chromosome abnormalities, but a firm diagnosis of this may often take up to two weeks. The main disadvantage of CVS is that it seems to carry a slightly greater risk of miscarriage than amniocentesis – around 1 per cent.

There have now been well over 60,000 CVS samples done around the world. These are recorded in a central data register in Philadelphia, and until recently there has been no evidence of any risk of this technique causing an abnormal baby. Unfortunately, in the event of a doubtful CVS result (particularly with some chromosomal problems), amniocentesis may be very occasionally required at a later date to confirm that the baby is normal.

Recently, there has been some evidence that CVS, done very early in pregnancy during the eighth or ninth week, may rarely carry a risk to the developing foetus. There have been a few reports of limb defects in the babies which have been born after CVS at this stage. Working in Oxford, Dr Firth and colleagues found that five babies were born with limb defects after 289 pregnancies underwent CVS at about eight weeks; quite similar data were confirmed independently by Dr Burton in 1992, in Chicago. He found that about 1 per cent of pregnancies subjected to early CVS ended with a baby being born with a limb abnormality. The reason for this is still unclear but doctors agree that for the time being caution is required before recommending very early CVS.

Other techniques of antenatal diagnosis

There are other important methods for detecting defects, which should be mentioned to complete the picture.

ULTRASOUND

Ultrasonic examination of babies is now, of course, common-place. It clearly ranks as one of the greatest advances in modern obstetrics for helping doctors to follow accurately the progress of a baby's growth in the womb. All available evidence shows that this is an extremely safe method.

In recent years, ultrasound has become even more accurate and the pictures through it have a better resolution. This means that a better view of the baby can be obtained and certain foetal defects can be diagnosed with it. Perhaps the three which are most important in earlier pregnancies are defects of the spinal cord, certain abnormalities of the head and defects of the heart. Unfortunately, even these are difficult to diagnose before about 18–19 weeks, which is very late to consider terminating pregnancy. Moreover, accurate diagnosis depends a good deal upon the operator's experience and in any case, not all routine ultrasound examinations will pick up all such defects, especially if they are small.

CHORDOCENTESIS

It is now possible to take blood from the baby in the womb. This is done by chordocentesis: after an injection of a little local anaesthetic, a needle is guided under ultrasound painlessly through the woman's abdominal wall into the uterus and then into the umbilical cord. This test can be done from seventeen weeks onwards. It requires special skill, but is safe, carrying no greater risk of miscarriage than CVS, i.e. about 1 per cent. It has the advantage over amniocentesis in that actual blood cells are retrieved, leading to rapid diagnosis of chromosome problems.

FOETOSCOPY

Some specialists in antenatal diagnosis insert a special telescope (known as a foetoscope), no thicker than a ball-point pen refill, into the uterus to look at the baby. Certain rare liver and skin diseases in the baby can be diagnosed this way. The examination is painless, though a little local anaesthetic is needed in the skin of the woman's abdomen.

HORMONE AND CHEMICAL TESTS

It has been known for quite a time that the babies of women with raised levels of a chemical called alpha-foetoprotein (AFP) are morely likely to have spinal cord defects such as spina bifida. This can be reliably detected in the fluid surrounding the baby after amniocentesis at around 12–14 weeks. AFP is also slightly raised in the woman's bloodstream in such pregnancies. However, the rise is small and blood tests alone are not reliable; amniocentesis must be done to confirm the diagnosis.

There has recently been a dramatic new use found for AFP blood testing. A team at St Bartholomew's Hospital in London has found that women carrying babies with Down's syndrome are more likely to have a lower-than-normal blood level of AFP as well as raised blood levels of HCG and a hormone called estriol. They found that if they tested levels of all three at once, they had a rapid screening test for Down's syndrome, which could be done at around sixteen weeks. This is important. At present in Britain, only about 15 per cent of all Down's syndrome babies are detected before birth. This screening test, if widely done in pregnancy, would certainly lead to more women at high risk subsequently going on to have amniocentesis and to the detection of at least 70 per cent of cases of Down's syndrome.

PREIMPLANTATION DIAGNOSIS

A very recent breakthrough is preimplantation diagnosis – the diagnosis of an embyronic defect between two and five days after fertilisation. This is a remarkable technique which prevents a pregnancy being affected by genetic disease. It was initially pioneered at Hammersmith Hospital, where the method was used to discover the sex of embryos (*see* Chapter 4) being transferred to the uterus in patients at risk of giving birth to boys with sex-linked disorders such as muscular dystrophy.

> Sheila knew that she might be a carrier of a genetic disease only after she had watched her fourteen-year-old brother die from muscular dystrophy. He had spent the last six years of his life, increasingly incapacitated, in a wheelchair. Sheila's blood test suggested that she might be a genetic carrier of the disease, which meant that any of her own sons could suffer a similar fate.
>
> Sheila married at nineteen. Her first two pregnancies were tested, found to be affected and were terminated at twenty-two weeks of pregnancy. Her husband could not cope with this, nor with Sheila's sadness and remorse. Their marriage broke up.
>
> Since then Sheila has remarried and has had three more

pregnancies. All three babies were diagnosed as having the disease and all have been aborted. Now neither she nor John, her husband, feel they can embark on another pregnancy and face the desolation of another termination. Both desperately want children. Preimplantation diagnosis would be a great benefit to them.

In families known to be at risk, the woman is given ovulatory drugs to encourage the ovaries to produce a large number of eggs. These are collected using IVF methods and fertilised with her husband's sperm. Each egg is then cultured in an IVF laboratory for two or three days until the embryos contain about eight cells. If both parents carry the same defective recessive gene, for example cystic fibrosis, 25 per cent of the embryos will be normal, 50 per cent will carry the defective gene and 25 per cent will be embryos which will be affected by the disease if allowed to become pregnancies. The invisible embryos are placed under a sophisticated microscope and one or two cells are removed microsurgically, using micromanipulators. The removal of cells, or biopsy, is very delicate with a structure of such small size. The microscope and micromanipulators need to be mounted on a rock-steady marble-topped table to kill vibration. In spite of having a really heavy table top, very slight vibration can be a real nuisance. For example, a heavy lorry driving up 30 or 40 yards away from the laboratory can induce movements which make the biopsy impossible.

Once a cell is removed from each embryo, the embryos are carefully replaced in culture tubes and returned to the culture oven pending a diagnosis. Each tube is, of course, carefully labelled so that it can be identified later. The cells are then individually broken up to liberate the DNA, the genetic message, from each of them. The DNA is then rapidly analysed using the PCR method (*see* p. 295). Within a matter of four to six hours, the scientists can tell whether each embryo carries one copy of the gene (in which case it will be an unaffected carrier like its parents), two copies of the gene (in which case it will be affected), or no copies of the gene, in which case it will be completely normal. Within minutes of completing the diagnosis, selected embryos can be returned to the mother's uterus, assuring that a future baby will be free of the disease in question.

The emotional advantages of such an approach are overwhelming. Until this technique was developed, couples at risk of having babies with fatal gene defects had to decide after amniocentesis or CVS whether to consider a termination of pregnancy. We have started to use it for couples who have had a baby die of a genetic disease already, and for those who are looking after an ill child affected by a gene defect. The technique overcomes the religious problems and moral qualms that many couples feel over abortion, and allows women to commence a pregnancy knowing it is free of their family's hereditary disease.

There are considerable problems with preimplantation diagnosis and much more research is needed before it can become widely available.

1. Preimplantation diagnosis currently requires IVF technology, with all the paraphernalia involved. IVF has a high failure rate in any one cycle of treatment, and there is only (in our hands) about a 30 per cent chance of conception. The treatment involves many hospital visits for ovulation induction and an operation for egg collection, and therefore is quite time-consuming for a working woman, or a mother looking after a child that is already sick. Moreoever there is the real risk of disappointment if the technique does not work.

2. To get the best chance of pregnancy we usually put two embryos, rather than one, back in the uterus, if available. This carries a small risk of twins, inconvenient for a family with an ill child already.

3. It is thought that removal of a cell from the embryo may slightly reduce its viability, and encourage a risk of miscarriage. So far, this has not been a significant problem, but we need to do more work to see whether the incidence of miscarriage is higher than after normal conception.

4. There is always the possibility that the diagnosis from a single cell may be flawed. Analysing the DNA from a single cell means that we are working absolutely at the cutting edge of what is possible, and is scientifically like flying a space shuttle.

Consequently, there is the risk that we might get the diagnosis wrong, and transfer an embryo to the uterus which turns out to be affected. A huge amount of research has been done on this over five years, and we calculate this risk to be no more than about 2 per cent. Nevertheless, couples undergoing this treatment are advised to have a back-up amniocentesis or CVS, if they wish, to confirm the diagnosis.

5. Lastly, there is the fear that by removing a cell from an embryo, we might damage the embryo and induce a new abnormality. Needless to say, a large number of experiments have been done in different animal species first and the technique seems to be completely safe. We also know that embryos are often missing one or two cells naturally, and there is no evidence at all that such embryos can give rise to a damaged child. However, at the time of writing, only eight babies have been born after this technique – all were entirely healthy – and many more pregnancies are needed before we can allow this treatment as a routine procedure.

The first baby after an embryo biopsy confirming it was free of cystic fibrosis was a little girl, conceived at Hammersmith and born in April 1992, in Burnley, Lancashire. She has an elder sister affected by cystic fibrosis and her birth offers great hopes to many thousands of families carrying various fatal genetic disorders.

SCREENING FOR FOETAL CELLS IN THE MOTHER'S BLOODSTREAM

Another experimental technique, currently being researched, involves screening maternal blood for cells from the developing baby, very early in pregnancy. The idea behind this comes from the knowledge that as the placenta starts to develop in very early pregnancy, it invades the mother's blood vessels in the uterus. Not surprisingly, some cells from the placenta break off and enter the mother's bloodstream. Consequently, a sample of blood, taken from a vein in the arm, will contain a few cells derived from the foetus. It is hoped that, in future, methods might be developed to extract these cells from the mother's blood, following which they could be tested by DNA analysis. There are a number of teething problems with the method for extracting the cells, but it is likely that in due course we will be able to screen babies in the uterus, without having to do either amniocentesis or CVS. This would avoid the risks associated with these two procedures.

An abnormal baby: choosing what to do

Once an abnormal baby has been detected, parents have a hard decision to make. Abortion is now widely accepted by our society, but is certainly not the right choice for everybody. Many people, particularly those who are deeply religious, believe that abortion is not a choice at all, and they will rightly refuse screening by amniocentesis or CVS.

However, it is not only those with deeply held religious views who do not accept abortion; some people simply feel that the baby has a right to life and that it is morally wrong to tamper with any pregnancy. They frequently point out that although there may be physical or mental impairment, many of these defects are quite compatible with a happy life. Children with Down's syndrome are an excellent example: given a stimulating environment, these children, who tend naturally to be happy, often develop remarkably well.

There is also no doubt that many women will refuse amniocentesis because of its lateness. As one woman said to me, 'I would have liked CVS earlier in this pregnancy had it been available, but I feel unable to go through amniocentesis now with this feeling that I would be destroying my living, moving child.' Another reason for refusing amniocentesis is the risk, however small, of miscarriage. Some women feel that they cannot accept even the remotest risk of damaging a normal baby.

The great majority of women who find that their babies are abnormal decide to terminate their pregnancies. This is partly because most of those who undergo antenatal testing have already made this decision if they are found to have a baby with a foetal abnormality. In spite of this, many women find that they are having to make a fresh decision when actually faced with the bad news. It may be an easier decision to make when the baby has a fatal condition, though there will still be feelings of guilt and deep responsibility. These feelings are heightened for most women when they are told that their babies have an abnormality such as Down's syndrome, because they recognise that such a baby may live to quite an advanced age.

Whatever the decision is, grief is an important process which needs to be gone through. Fortunately, clinics now are more supportive and many have counselling services, though often these still fall well short of ideal.

Getting the test result

Finding out that your baby is abnormal is a horrible, numbing shock. The mutual support of both partners can be very important when you get the news and also when you have to make decisions. In my view, the man should always be encouraged to be with the woman during the amniocentesis or ultrasound examination, and certainly when returning to the antenatal clinic to get test results. Unfortunately (and, I think, wrongly), some women are given these results by telephone. I think it better that they should be handled face to face, with the doctor and both partners present. Male partners should also, in my opinion, recognise that they will be needed much more at home following a 'bad' diagnosis.

Although sharing the grief may be important, men and women react differently to termination. The experience itself cannot be entirely shared – after all, the baby grows and moves inside the woman, not the man. Of course the knowledge of a defective baby can draw some couples closer together. However, no matter how shocked they are, men usually find it easier to cope with a termination, for example, immersing themselves in their work. Most women take longer in their grieving, not least because of the physical changes that a pregnancy has demanded of their bodies. The fact that a woman may still be mourning while her partner is apparently remote can drive a couple apart. It may also be very important for a woman to find other people in whom she can confide, perhaps a close friend or relative. This may also be extremely helpful when deciding whether to terminate or not.

The medical profession has not always been very good in this situation. Up to now there has been remarkably little support for couples taking these momentous decisions, for the bereaved couple who have undergone a termination, or the couple who have decided to keep a damaged child. There is no doubt that parents, especially women, are put under huge pressure by our society, which finds it difficult to accept, understand or tolerate handicap. There is an assumption that a couple, and especially the woman, will rapidly 'get over it'. Some doctors and nurses are even insensitive enough to imply that 'another pregnancy' will soon make a couple forget the unhappiness of this one. Such attitudes are becoming less common, and fortunately there is the slowly growing recognition that people need much more support and counselling.

There is also too little sensitively written information. Too much has been published that contains only medical facts and easy solutions (usually written, I fear, by doctors). Alternatively, there are one or two very angry books which are virulently feminist; these, I think, would be damaging and disturbing for most women facing these questions. One book I strongly recommend is The Tentative Pregnancy by Barbara Katz Rothman (see p. 347). This offers sensitive and compassionate advice to women considering whether to undergo amniocentesis and termination of pregnancy.

CHAPTER FIFTEEN

Manipulating our Genesis: Ethics and Politics

Few areas of human activity have caused more debate in recent years than the developments in human reproduction. IVF and related areas have had an extraordinary profile, because in this century, for the first time, humans have had truly effective means to manipulate and control the beginnings of life.

The use of medical resources

The world is facing a crisis in providing adequate medical care. The increasing price of high technology medicine and the cost of caring for ageing populations threaten health care in richer countries. In the developing world, basic, essential medical care is often hopelessly deficient. In both kinds of society people have greater expectations from medical services than can be easily provided. These problems are particularly serious in hospital medicine, the most expensive of medical services and, incidentally, where reproductive medicine tends to be based. When people are suffering from potentially fatal illness, or experiencing such pain that they are unable to work, or have inadequate access to health care screening which may detect potentially fatal disease and lead to its effective treatment, how can infertility treatments be remotely justified? Ironically, infertility treatments would seem to be the last requirement of humankind. After all, the most serious problem our planet faces is an expanding human population, a deteriorating environment and limited energy resources. Can the treatment of infertility be justified when a substantial percentage of the Earth's inhabitants face starvation?

Nobody dies from infertility. Yet diseases affecting human fertility and reproduction are serious because they cause great hardship to so many individuals and are destructive to vital components of human society. Human infertility is such a serious problem in various ways in different societies that it surely justifies adequate provision of treatment.

The high incidence (10 per cent) of infertility has important implications for those providing health care. In Britain, there are about 11.7 million females between the ages of sixteen and forty-four, i.e. of reproductive age. If we assume, at the very least, that half of this population is likely some time to want children, and if we assume that roughly 10 per cent is infertile, there must be at least 600,000 infertile women in the UK. In the United States, it is reasonable to presume that at least 2–3 million people are infertile.

Infertility, and the deep distress it causes, is not a new phenomenon. It is no coincidence that infertility features so commonly in the Bible. Remarkably, three out of the four matriarchs, Sarah, Rebecca and Rachel, were infertile. Genesis eloquently depicts Rachel's grief at finding herself sterile: 'Give me children, else I am as good as dead'; the biblical account also dwells on her husband's anger at her complaint, showing the rift developing between husband and wife. Infertility always seems to have been a private complaint causing deep shame; for example, Hannah's infertility and subsequent private prayer in the temple leads the High Priest, Eli, to accuse her of being drunk. This stigma of infertility has continued until modern times, and is still especially severe in many countries of the developing world where for a woman to be infertile is the ultimate shame. In many Moslem societies, infertility is adequate grounds for divorce. Infertile women are very insecure and quite frequently may be abandoned by their spouse. The biggest drive for fertility is most frequently found in societies that perhaps can least afford to raise children. In the rural Western Province of Kenya where, to say the least, living conditions are extremely primitive, the average family size is eight and most families when questioned would like twelve. Here infertility (or even contraception) carries a serious stigma. For poorer people, living in an underprivileged society, a family (and more particularly a large family) represents a considerable degree of wealth and security. Wealth, because children can soon contribute to the family economy and security because parents, in their later years, can be cared for by their children. These factors have traditionally been most important in farming communities; childlessness in such a society carries very serious consequences.

In Western society, publicity surrounding IVF and other similar reproductive techniques has at least heightened awareness of how serious being infertile really is. It has brought it out in the open. But even in our society, the experience of infertility causes most couples anxiety, leading frequently to anger, loss of self-esteem, guilt, and feelings of deep frustration. Of course, not all couples react the same way and many rapidly come to terms with it. However, for the majority, these early feelings often grow worse, with isolation from friends and family, lack of sexual satisfaction or impotence, depression and feelings of grief or bereavement. Occasionally, depression can be relatively severe, with disruption of both home and job.

Consequently, whilst infertility does not cause major physical disease and whilst the diseases which cause infertility are not usually life-threatening, the disability and pain which infertility causes is worthy of the most serious concern. The problems caused by intractable infertility are often every bit as significant as the problems caused by arthritis of the hip or even serious lung disease. Moreover, infertility is probably more common than either of those two serious chronic conditions but fewer resources are devoted to its treatment.

PROVISION OF INFERTILITY TREATMENTS

Even in most developed countries, provision of comprehensive care for infertility treatments is haphazard. Infertility is generally not regarded as serious and provision in the public sector is limited. In most parts of the United States, infertility investigation and treatment are widely available but only in the private sector. In America, insurance companies vary in their attitude towards high-technology treatments such as in vitro fertilisation, but may provide cover for a number of attempts at IVF. In general, procedures such as laparoscopy or tubal surgery are covered, as may be induction of ovulation. Things are similar in many European countries; the state provides some basic care but IVF has to be purchased by the consumer. In Israel, all infertility treatments including IVF are available in the public sector. This is a significant factor in Israel's relatively high standing in research into human reproduction and infertility. However, in a hard-pressed economy like Israel's, the public sector has become increasingly poorly funded and some patients seek private treatment, particularly IVF, largely because they prefer the comfort, privacy and perceived better success rates in the private sector.

In Britain, the National Health Service (NHS) offers basic care for infertile patients. This free treatment is remarkably patchy and frequently depends on the special interest of a local consultant. Dedicated infertility clinics are relatively new in Britain. A recent survey showed that, of the 200 health districts in England and Wales, only one-quarter could offer tubal microsurgery and well under half had facilities for ovarian scanning by ultrasound. Only about one-third returned hormone test results within the same menstrual cycle as when blood sampling was undertaken. Under 10 per cent offered any infertility counselling and donor insemination was available (with usually considerable waiting lists) in only a handful of places. There were only seven health districts which could truly be said to be providing a comprehensive infertility service (excluding IVF). At the time of this survey, there were only two IVF clinics in the UK wholly funded by the NHS. Since then, one of these has largely closed its doors, though a few other clinics have achieved partial funding to a limited extent from the NHS. Waiting lists for IVF are disgracefully long. In spite of the government's Patient Charter, the pledge that no

NHS patient would wait for longer than two years for hospital treatment, IVF patients frequently wait four years, or even more. This is particularly demoralising for women because their fertility declines with age. It means that many couples get treatment which is too late to be of help, and others none at all.

THE SELECTION OF PATIENTS

Which patients the doctor should treat is another serious source of controversy. In the private sector, the decision is easy and most couples find that they can buy treatment without great difficulty and without too many questions about their 'suitability' for parenthood. In the public sector the selection of patients, particularly for IVF, remains very problematic. This issue has been prominent in Britain. Nearly all NHS units limit treatments to some degree. The commonest criterion is the age of the female partner. Most refuse to treat any woman over forty years old; normally, the upper age limit is set lower than this, at between thirty-five and thirty-eight. Purely in terms of applying resources to the couples most likely to benefit, the harsh policy of limiting treatment to younger women can be justified. This is formal policy in Denmark, where a woman must be under thirty-seven years old to enter the waiting list for IVF and treatment is barred after forty years of age. This is very hard for older couples to accept.

Another criterion frequently used is marriage, or at least a stable partnership. In South Australia, artificial fertilisation procedures are only allowed under the Reproductive Technology Act, 1988, for 'married' couples. A married couple is defined as one that has cohabited continuously for at least five years. The State of Victoria, Australia, enacted the Infertility (Medical Procedures) Act in 1984 which provided that in vitro fertilisation was permissible for married couples only. Under this Act, pretreatment counselling was made compulsory. In Denmark, a woman must be in a stable relationship for at least three years before treatment is permitted. Whilst there is no formal law in Italy, a working party of gynaecologists agreed a code of practice there in 1984 which limits the treatment to married couples only. In Norway things are much stricter and couples are asked to sign a declaration that they are married before treatment. Spanish law is much less rigid. In 1988, the Spanish government agreed that IVF might be made available to any woman, married or not. In Britain there is no legal requirement to be married, or even to be in a stable relationship. In practice, though, only a very few physicians seem to be prepared to offer IVF for single women who have no male partner; those that are are limited to the private sector.

A further restriction is sometimes made to those who already have a child, or children. In Britain, with a few exceptions, NHS units do not offer IVF to those couples who already have one child from the existing relationship. At Hammersmith, we have generally limited free IVF to those who have no more than one child in the existing relationship; in practice we have found this policy rather invidious and, inevitably, some of our patients are now returning for their third or even fourth IVF child. In Denmark there is a stipulation that a couple must be childless before treatment; nor may they have any adopted children.

In Britain, it is frequently found that individual doctors, both general practitioners and specialists, are reluctant to offer treatments to couples from very poor economic circumstances, or those who are unemployed. In my view, in many ways these couples are, if anything, more deserving of treatment because a child offers fulfilment in one aspect of their hard lives. Most of these decisions certainly seem to aim to ration resources. Formal restrictions mostly apply in Denmark, Norway, and Australia, where there is some government funding for the treatment, or for the drugs which are used. However, in France, Belgium and Spain, the state offers social security funds or public funding of IVF and yet there are no formal rules about which patients may receive treatment. One has the feeling that the restrictions which are generally agreed in individual countries say as much about attitudes of society and doctors as they do about resources.

In my view it seems wrong to ration IVF, or indeed any

other infertility treatment, on the basis of an arbitrary cut-off point such as age. Unless it is clear that the patient is so old that there is no realistic chance of success, why should a patient have less access to treatment? Indeed, even when there is no chance at all of producing a successful pregnancy, treatment may still be justified. Some women benefit from going through a treatment and failing. This may help them to come to terms with their infertility, knowing that they have done everything possible to achieve pregnancy. Whilst counselling should be aimed at preventing or reducing unnecessary treatment cycles, occasionally a failure may be far more therapeutic, allowing a woman and her partner to enter a period of bereavement and mourning, with possible resolution and healing afterwards.

TREATING SINGLE WOMEN AND LESBIAN COUPLES

There has been considerable discussion about infertility treatments for single women who have no intention of living with a male partner or those single women living with another woman, possibly in a lesbian relationship. Doctors are very reluctant to offer such women treatment, though they find it difficult to provide a rational reason for refusal. Anecdotal evidence is occasionally produced suggesting that babies born to lesbian mothers may in some way be disadvantaged and may suffer from the lack of a father figure as 'role-model'. Some prominent feminist writers are incensed by this attitude – typical is Ms Gena Corea: 'Physicians and other pharmacrats, the vast majority of whom are white, male and middle to upper class, choose which women are endowed with the right to bear test-tube babies.' One could point out to Ms Corea that many doctors, neither white, male, nor even upper class, may have some misgivings about offering very expensive and difficult technology if they feel there is a real risk to the welfare of any offspring. Regrettably, IVF raises many emotions and too many people on both sides of 'moral' arguments are too ready to shout opinions.[39] What is needed is more research to decide if children from certain 'family' origins do run greater risks during later development.

The status of the human embryo

Many people believe that human life begins at conception and that to tamper with or damage a human embryo is nothing short of causing the destruction of a human being. Some go as far as to say that to experiment with human embryos is a kind of Nazi endeavour. Often, people who believe this, point to the Helsinki Medical Declaration which states that doctors must respect all human life and do their best to preserve it. I do not pretend to have an unbiased view, but there is a strong case against this opinion.

First, if 'life' does begin at conception, presumably all that precedes fertilisation is not 'alive'. This argument suggests that the egg is not 'human life' or that sperm are not alive. This is palpably untrue. Moreover, this argument implies that, magically, there is a single moment when that which is not human, and therefore sacred, is suddenly invested with sanctity. This argument is difficult to sustain. If life 'begins' at fertilisation, we still have to define a point when life starts. As we have seen from Chapter 1, fertilisation is a continuous process, taking many hours. If life truly begins at fertilisation, does the point of absolute protection commence with the time when sperm become attached to the egg, penetrate it, or when cell division starts to occur? If the latter, at what point of cell division, for the first cell division is part of a continuous process.

The truth is surely, that life is really part of a continuum, and that as the embryo develops, it becomes increasingly more

[39] I have not addressed the feminist objections to embryo research in this book, which may or may not be regarded as 'moral arguments'. Relatively extreme feminists seem to believe that this research is done by men to manipulate women. This seems to denigrate women and fails to credit them with any intelligence. In my own group of about fifteen scientists, only three are men.

'human'. Thus, for example, we do not have a funeral service for an early miscarriage, and certainly removal of an early foetus from the uterus is not regarded as murder in European law. There are good precedents for this way of thinking. In the thirteenth century, St Thomas Aquinas, that great Catholic theologian, argued that the flesh (in Latin, *cara*) is formed at conception, but that the soul (*anima*) enters the embryo at some later time. He regarded a complete human as only being in existence once the process of ensoulment had been established. This idea follows an important Western tradition. In ancient Greece, Aristotle argued that the soul was only established a good time after conception. Jewish tradition, from which so much of Christian thinking is derived, suggests that the embryo is '*Meoh b'almoh*' – mere fluid – until forty days after conception. Jews do not therefore regard early abortion as the taking of human life, but abortion becomes increasingly grave the further human development has gone. For Jews, as in current English law, the child is not offered full legal protection until the head of the foetus is actually born.

There are good biological reasons for refusing to accept that the early developing embryo is a full human being. Firstly, it certainly is not a unique individual, because twinning can spontaneously occur up to fourteen days after fertilisation. Secondly, the great majority of human embryos – around 80 per cent, as we have seen – are simply shed after conception. Nature herself does not regard the embryo as sacrosanct. Thirdly, the human embryo up to fourteen days has no independent means of survival; it has not implanted yet in the mother's womb, and only has a potential for being human, just as any one of many hundreds of million sperm may give rise to a unique human being. Finally, before fourteen days, the human embryo is so small that it is invisible to the naked eye. Of course, smallness does not preclude humanity, but at this stage it has no organs, no nervous system, no brain and therefore no sensibility, sensation or consciousness.

This lack of a central nervous system does, I think, offer a real pointer as to the status of the embryo. We do already have an accepted definition of life and death. In the case of kidney, liver, or heart transplantation, the law allows and society accepts that we may remove these organs from a body for surgical transplantation, providing that the body is dead and there is no higher neurological activity. Death is defined as the moment of brain death – the heart of the donor may be beating, but 'life' can only be sustained by breathing apparatus. The donor is 'brain dead'. Perhaps therefore it is logical and ethical to regard the beginning of human 'life' as when there is an indication of brain life.

It is this kind of thinking which, I believe, most influenced the Warnock Commission which was set up to pronounce on various aspects of the status of the embryo. Warnock ruled that the first fourteen days after fertilisation were a separate phase of human development and that it would be reasonable to conduct studies on embryos for human benefit before this time.

The benefits of embryo research

There is no doubt that embryo research can be of great benefit.

INFERTILITY

Research with human embryos is crucial if we are to improve the comparatively poor results of infertility treatment. IVF itself would not have been possible without embryo research. Indeed, the first babies born – sacred human life – could not have existed without this research. Human embryos had to be studied after fertilisation outside the body to ensure that such an artificial environment does not cause any birth defects.

Regrettably, IVF remains one of the least successful of all fertility treatments. We do not understand, for example, why the culture conditions we use in the laboratory result in only about 15 per cent of healthy-looking embryos successfully implanting after transfer to the uterus. Treatment of male infertility is even more unreliable. We saw in Chapter 8 that only about 10 per cent of infertile men have a treatable defect. New treatments, such as sperm injection into the egg (*see* p. 216) require the scientist to ensure that embryos generated by such methods are normal, and cannot give rise to damaged babies. Such work, though started in animals, must be completed using human embryos because animals do not always suffer the same birth defects.

GENETIC DISEASE

Embryo research is also vital if we are to improve our understanding and handling of genetic diseases. I have already indicated that these represent one of the greatest unsolved problems in modern medicine. Many, if not most, of these diseases are unique to humans and cannot be tackled or properly investigated using animal eggs and sperm. Although some research can be done looking at other cells in culture, it is the early embryo which goes wrong, and it is this which requires closest study.

A very good example of the value of embryo research is the recent advance of preimplantation diagnosis. Without this research, some healthy babies in families that had already lost a child would not have existed. In the previous chapter, we saw that CVS is generally more acceptable than amniocentesis in the antenatal diagnosis of abnormal babies, because this can occur so much earlier. Nevertheless, this still leaves a couple facing a decision regarding abortion. Preimplantation diagnosis, on embryos before pregnancy actually commences, is an attractive alternative. It is ethically desirable, because it avoids abortion of a fully formed pregnancy.

There are, however, a number of problems with preimplantation diagnosis which still require careful investigation. One is whether, by taking a cell away for examination from a human embryo, scientists might actually cause a defect. Another is whether examination of a single cell from the embryo is really representative and completely reliable. One very important spin-off from this work has been the development of methods to examine human embryos in considerable detail. Apart from the value of DNA itself, this research has started to demonstrate that certain defects actually occur after conception. We are therefore much closer to understanding these defects, and possibly how they might be prevented.

As an example, one recent important find has been the discovery of methods to paint individual chromosomes in embryonic cells. Dr Joy Delhanty, at University College, London, has pioneered much of this research which can be used to detect the sex of an embryo in cases of sex-linked disease, or to establish whether certain chromosomal defects are present. There are very important applications of this technology. They include the avoidance of pregnancies with Down's syndrome, and possibly improving the reproductive ability of older women starting a pregnancy for the first time. Had embryo research been banned in Britain, this valuable knowledge would have been lost.

Unfortunately, there has been a huge campaign conducted against embryo research. This has delayed important, valuable scientific advances because units have been reluctant to invest hard-pressed funds and academic energy into an area which might have been prematurely banned by hasty legislation.

MISCARRIAGE

A third reason for embryo research is miscarriage. In Britain alone, over 100,000 women each year are admitted to hospital with threatened or incomplete miscarriages. Leaving aside the huge financial cost, there is a huge emotional cost which even doctors are only just beginning to understand. A miscarriage also involves considerable health risks and quite a few women remain infertile afterwards; others may develop painful symptoms of chronic pelvic infection.

In 80 per cent of cases, we have very little idea what really has caused a miscarriage. We know that most miscarried pregnancies arise from abnormal embryos, but we have very little idea of what causes those abnormal embryos in the first place, and what measures might prevent those abnormalities. Application of the work done by Dr Delhanty is very likely to have a major impact in this area. There can be little doubt that human embryo research is still essential if we are to make any serious progress in this field.

IMPLANTATION AND ECTOPIC PREGNANCY

A fourth reason for embryo research is to understand how embryos implant. We know that the majority of human embryos actually fail to implant in the uterus, and are lost. Some are abnormal, of course, but by no means all. If we knew how human embryos implant, and what chemical messages pass between the embryos and uterus, we would be in a better position to understand miscarriage, contraception, ectopic pregnancy and early development. Ectopic pregnancy is a dangerous emergency. In Jamaica, about 1 in 15 pregnancies are ectopic; ectopics, especially in countries with limited health care, are one of the most common causes of women dying in pregnancy. Yet ectopic pregnancy is a mystifying condition; we simply do not know why so many pregnancies implant inside the tube. Ectopic pregnancy is virtually unknown in any animal species apart from man. There seems to be something peculiar about human implantation which predisposes women to this important problem. Currently scientists are starting to grow human embryos with uterine lining cells to evaluate some of these problems.

CANCER

It may seem extraordinary to suggest that embryo research could give insights into the understanding and treatment of cancer. None the less, several researchers are pursuing investigations in this area. Every cell in the body carries a group of genes called *oncogenes* – the 'housekeeping' genes that control each cell's growth and division. Cancer is basically a disease in which some cells start to divide very rapidly and abnormally. If we knew what goes wrong with the genes controlling cell

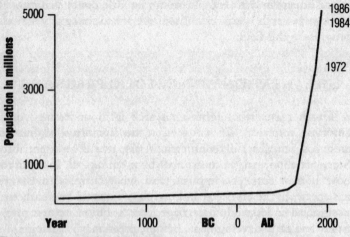

The burgeoning population of the world.

division, we might have sufficient insight to work out new treatments. The early embryonic cells, which provide an ideal model for the action of oncogenes, are in many ways perfect for this kind of study.

Contraception

The graph above dramatically shows the world's burgeoning population. This has grown frighteningly, although many estimates suggest that the rate of growth may now be slowing. Nevertheless, the United Nations states that, by the year 2100, it will reach 10,185 million, twice what it is now. Other estimates put it at considerably more than this. Whatever the speed of growth, it is clear that the populations of Europe and North American will remain relatively static, and that the main burden of this huge increase in humanity will be borne by the poorest nations who can least afford to support it. It is this threat, above all, which has stimulated the World Health Organization's attempts to improve existing methods of contraception.[40]

Most current methods of contraception are short of ideal. Most have side-effects and some have potential dangers. Sterilisation, both male and female, is largely irreversible and therefore often unacceptable. A new approach is needed. Work is in progress to look at methods of immunising people against an early developing pregnancy. Other alternatives are substances which interfere with fertilisation or with early embryonic growth. Embryo research is vital in the investigation of all of these different methods, not least because it will be essential to ensure that such methods do not cause damage to an embryo which 'slips through the contraceptive net', in the event of contraceptive failure. While an occasional failure of a contraceptive method is just acceptable, this would not be so if a deformed or damaged baby was born as a result of contraceptive usage.

To be fair, the graphs may be too gloomy. Incorrect predictions of catastrophe are not new. In 1798 Thomas Malthus calculated that Britain's population would rise from its then 7 million to 112 million by the year 1900. He also thought that, by 1900, food supplies in Britain would support no more than 35 million people, and he forecast famine or enforced mass emigration. Then there was no solution to his perceived dilemma as the population in the rest of the world would have expanded in a similar way; emigration would not have helped. We know now that Malthus was wrong. Even without contraception, British population growth did not meet his worst expectations but slowed substantially. The factors which brought this about were largely social. There were great improvements in living standards, in diet, in social equality, in

[40] In this respect at least, the British government has shown commendable wisdom. It provides more money for contraceptive programmes and research than nearly any other country, and is a leading contributor to WHO's human reproduction programme. Contrast the stance of the USA under Presidents Reagan and Bush. They have consistently refused more than the most meagre help. For the richest country in the world to be so remote from the Earth's needs is a matter of the greatest concern. Hopefully this stance will change with President Clinton.

education and in political and social stability. The death rate decreased with improvements in health care and the prevention of disease. All this led to what has been termed 'population maturation', with a fall in birth-rate in developed countries: people no longer felt the need to have large families because so many more of their children were surviving.

Things are different in developing countries now. While the introduction of Western-style medicine has caused death rates to fall rapidly, the birth-rate remains high. The difference is that, in the West, the death-rate came down gradually over 200 years, and the birth-rate responded by falling approximately fifty years later. In developing countries, the drop in the death-rate has been too sudden and dramatic for us to expect to see a corresponding fall in birth-rate.[41] Moreover, most developing countries remain pitifully poor and relatively unstable. Consequently, we are yet to witness the effect of population maturation in the developing world.

One natural method of contraception is breastfeeding. While a woman is lactating, her periods stop and she seldom ovulates. Women of the Kung tribe from the Kalahari, who marry very young yet use no form of contraception nor abortion, breastfeed their babies by continuous suckling for at least three years after birth. This provides an ideal way of limiting family size and they have an average of fewer than five babies per family. You may remember Mrs McNaught, mentioned in Chapter 1. She gave birth, in separate pregnancies, to twelve boys and ten girls in twenty-two years. After each pregnancy, her doctor gave her injections to stop her breast milk. Perhaps if she had breastfed her babies, she might not be in the *Guinness Book of Records*.

WHO points out that we should encourage far more

---

[41] It is a horrifying paradox to consider how Western medicine and attitudes have, in certain ways, caused very difficult problems in the developing world. A few years ago, I was in a children's care centre in rural India. There were perhaps 300 orphans standing around in a primitive playing field, all between the ages of five and seven; none was the size of my own four-year-old child. It suddenly occurred to me that, were vaccination and antibiotics not available, few of these children would be alive.

breastfeeding, especially in developing countries. Cow's milk or powdered substitutes, given in bottles, are a potent cause of serious disease and fatal diarrhoea in hot countries, where infections cannot be controlled. Pope John Paul II, in his *Humanae Vitae* has insisted that contraception is wrong except where 'natural cycles' are used. This causes great difficulties for the 800 million Catholics in the world. The Church could do much by encouraging breastfeeding. Less insistence on sexual abstinence and more emphasis on lactation might cut birth-rates and ensure fewer infant deaths from gastroenteritis and similar causes. [42]

Donor eggs, sperm and embryos

Another major ethical issue concerns donation of this unique human material. Many of the arguments have already been addressed in Chapter 12. A number of important questions are raised.

THE DONORS

What is the possibility that donors may subsequently regret giving their unique genetic 'material', and what kind of advice and counselling should be available? How should donors be selected and what screening procedures are permissible; what happens if a donor is found to have AIDS, for example? Should he or she be told of this impending fatal disease, and if not, what protection can be offered to others who might come into contact with the donor? Should donors receive payment, or should they only be allowed to act as donors through pure altruism? How many times is it permissible to use a sperm

[42] Of course, it should not be thought that breastfeeding is a highly reliable method of contraception. Probably 5–10 per cent of women continue to ovulate at least some of the time while feeding. The amount of suckling is important: once the baby is having supplementary feeds, breastfeeding should not be used alone if another pregnancy is really not wanted.

donor, knowing that many half-brothers or sisters may be produced? Does the donor have any right to know the outcome of the act of donation, or to whom the egg, sperm or embryo was given? Does the donor have any legal liability in this respect, in the event of an offspring tracing the donor subsequently? Do the donor's close relatives have a right to know that they may have a half-sister or brother or other close relative as a result of the act of donation? To what extent is it acceptable to put an egg donor at risk by the use of ovarian stimulation and operative egg collection? Can an infertile IVF patient's 'spare' eggs be used for donation, when the recipient may get pregnant but the donor not, during the cycle of treatment?

THE CHILD

Do children have the right to know of their origins and have a right to trace their genetic parents? May children be damaged by the knowledge that they are not genetically related to one or both of their parents? What are the dangers in keeping acts of donation secret from any resulting child?

THE RECIPIENTS

Who are to be regarded as suitable persons to receive eggs, sperm or embryos and who should be responsible for their selection? Should recipients be allowed or advised to keep their treatment a secret from the child, and what effect may this have on the family? Does donation have an adverse effect on a married couple's relationship? If infertile women have a right to have infertility treatment and egg or sperm donation, does this right extend to lesbian couples or single women who may also want to be mothers?

EFFECT ON SOCIETY

What risks are there of consanguinity – i.e. does the fact that there may be a number of half-brothers and half-sisters around mean that there is a risk of them unwittingly meeting and marrying?[43] Does donation of eggs and sperm cause some risk to the institution of marriage – is it, for example, a form of adultery?

Surrogacy

Some infertile women have no uterus, possibly as a result of disease or hysterectomy. Surrogacy is one possible solution; another woman can have a baby for the woman who is childless, giving it up at birth. There are two versions of surrogacy. The surrogate mother's own eggs may be fertilised naturally, possibly after artificial insemination from the adopting male partner. The other version is when a fertilised embryo, produced by an egg taken from the adopting mother after IVF, is transferred for 'incubation' into the surrogate mother's uterus.

Surrogacy is not new. In the Bible, Sarah was infertile, and she suggested to her husband Abram that he have a child by Hagar, her Egyptian handmaiden, which she might then adopt. She argues to Abram that 'perhaps I may obtain children by her . . .'[44] (Genesis 16:2). Ishmael is born as a result, and followers of Genesis will well know the trouble which this first surrogacy agreement subsequently caused. Surrogate arrange-

---

[43] Dr Curie-Cohen, writing in the *American Journal of Human Genetics* 1980, calculates that the risk of consanguinity inadvertently occurring as a result of donor programmes in the USA is small – a consanguineous relationship would occur once in only every 4.5 years. This is indeed a low risk, but still too high for religious authorities.

[44] The Hebrew of this passage is most instructive and perceptive. The literal translation of what Sarah actually says is, 'Perhaps I may be builded up through her . . .' Sarah is implying that she is of low esteem, and that this esteem may be built up if she has a child.

ments have always interested society, and there is little doubt that various forms of private surrogacy have always been practised. Our recent ability to manipulate reproduction has reawoken interest in surrogacy, which has been the subject of intense press interest. The pros and cons have perplexed many good lawyers and doctors; moral philosophy and moral philosophers – virtually a moribund speciality practised by a dying breed of academics – has been given the kiss of life by this recent flurry of activity.

There are a number of serious arguments against surrogacy. First, a baby born to a surrogate mother has, in reality, three parents. People who criticise surrogate arrangements argue that this could cause great confusion with family values, and cause anguish to the growing child. The baby may, for various reasons, be rejected by the adopting parents and the surrogate mother may be appalled at the consequences for her natural offspring. She may feel compelled to look after a baby she did not intend to keep. More important, there is a very real risk to the surrogate mother, whose attitude to her baby may change radically with advancing pregnancy, or after the baby is born. Jonathan Glover, the Oxford philosopher, has written: 'If she does decide to keep the baby, this may shatter the expectations of the couple who were expecting the child and leaves the father thinking that *his* child has been taken away.' If a law court enforces the surrogacy arrangement, as in the famous case against Mary Beth Whitehead (the surrogate mother who was initially forced to give up her child in the United States), the bearing mother may feel devastated.

To my mind surrogate arrangements are dangerous, particularly when sums of money have changed hands. Indeed, in Britain, commercial surrogacy has been illegal since 1987. There is no doubt, also, that the risk to the bearing mother's emotional health must be very great, particularly if a degree of psychological bonding between mother and pregnancy has occurred by the time of birth. There may also be severe problems if the baby is born with a chance genetic defect. The infant may be rejected by all the parents involved. Another major problem may occur if the surrogate mother becomes ill during the pregnancy. It is not clear who is morally and legally responsible for the effect on the mother and for her medical care. Nor is it clear whether a surrogate mother, intending to give up a baby after birth, is legally liable for any effects on someone else's genetic child if she does not look after her own health during pregnancy. Who is responsible, for example, if she smokes heavily or drinks excessively during the pregnancy?

Male pregnancy

IVF techniques have opened all sorts of extraordinary possibilities. There is no doubt that a male pregnancy is now technically feasible. Indeed, some laboratory attempts at this have already been made in small mammals and baboons. The embryo and its surrounding placental tissue are highly invasive and a human embryo could implant almost anywhere. Given the right hormonal environment, an embryo could be implanted in the abdominal cavity of a man, where it could grow until viability.[45] Because men do not have a uterus or a vagina, a normal delivery would be out of the question. The resulting pregnancy would need to be delivered by a form of Caesarean section, by surgically removing the baby from the abdomen near term.

Many people have been surprised that there might actually be serious indications for deliberating inducing an abdominal pregnancy in a man. Professor Walters, a very serious obstetri-

[45] Not just fanciful thinking; I have delivered three abdominal pregnancies, before the days of ultrasound, when diagnosis in advance was much more difficult. The first was in the dead of winter; I was in training in an isolated maternity unit in Essex. Because labour did not progress, I started a Caesarean section at 2.30 in the morning. Opening the abdomen, I could see the baby which at first I thought was in the bladder. I could not make the anatomy out at all, so telephoned my boss from the operating theatre. He lived eight miles away and was completely snowed in: 'I've no idea – you're on your own, Bob!' A live girl (7 pounds) eventually came out but I only stopped the extensive bleeding, where the placenta had implanted over the blood vessels in the pelvis, with great difficulty. I am pleased to say the mother survived my inexpert surgery.

cian from Australia, has argued that such a procedure could be considered in the case of a male transexual, who is living as a woman in a stable partnership with another man. Many transsexuals are known to have the strongest mothering instincts, and feel deprived because they cannot have babies. This technology could theoretically be used to allow them to have children. Another indication, which has been suggested in the lay and medical press, has been for a pregnancy in the case of two male homosexuals living in permanent partnership.

Perhaps the best medical indication might be for the treatment of women suffering from testicular feminisation syndrome. In this curious and fairly rare disorder, a person who is genetically male, carrying the normal male complement of chromosomes, is born without a uterus or ovaries, but with the rudiments of a vagina and normal female feelings. They are to all intents and purposes women and, following puberty, undergo normal breast development spontaneously. Oddly, people suffering from testicular feminisation are typically very good-looking women, and many of the patients I have known with this genetic problem are particularly attractive. One I know became an Olympic athlete of some distinction, but, after chromosome testing, she had a hard time persuading the Olympic officials that she was truly a woman. Women with testicular feminisation marry in the usual way and are able to have an entirely normal, pleasurable sexual relationship with orgasm. Unfortunately, because they have no uterus or ovaries, babies are impossible. Abdominal implantation of an embryo would be the only treatment possible for them. Such treatment has also been requested from time to time from caring husbands of infertile women who have been made infertile following severe uterine disease and hysterectomy. Several men have asked whether it might be possible for them to have the baby on their wife's behalf.

In the *Sun* newspaper, 28 May 1992, a photograph of a pregnant man was carried. Accompanied by a photograph and massive headlines, Carlo, the Pregnant Man, from the Philippines, was quoted: '"I can feel my boy kicking", says miracle Carlo.' The father, an army officer who refused to be identified, was quoted as saying, 'Of course, who would not be proud?' A subsequent issue of this newspaper, in much smaller type, admitted that Carlo's pregnancy was a hoax.

I think it rather doubtful that men will try to usurp the biological role of women, and attempt to have babies. First, few men would wish to take the massive female hormone treatment necessary to create the right environment for a pregnancy. Most men seem threatened by the perturbing idea that they might grow breasts. Second, abdominal pregnancy is a form of ectopic pregnancy (see Chapter 13) and carries severe risks of sudden catastrophic haemorrhage, particularly when a pregnancy is well advanced. Third, abdominal surgery to deliver a baby is not an especially appealing idea for most males, particularly when it might involve themselves rather than their partners. Nor do I think it all that likely that men will tolerate morning sickness and waiting in antenatal clinics. I suspect that women will continue to call the shots when it comes to reproducing our beleaguered species.

The artificial womb

In his witty, futuristic novel, Brave New World (1933), Aldous Huxley abolished birth. At Central Hatchery and Conditioning Centres all humans were conceived in test-tubes after cloning, and grown on conveyor belts outside the womb in racks of test-tubes. Two hundred and seventy days after fertilisation, following various conditioning processes to make them suitable for particular jobs needed by society, they were decanted. Huxley's masterpiece has had a profound effect on our thinking about ectogenesis, or conception outside the womb, and I believe the shocks in Brave New World continue to reverberate. The concept of an artificial womb horrified his society and still contributes to some extent to our suspicion of modern reproductive technology.

The world's first test-tube baby was not in reality born until forty-five years later, but this birth awakened many of the antagonistic feelings that people had about extrauterine conception. How close are we today in producing complete gestation outside the body?

One of the basic problems about extrauterine conception is that once the mammalian embryo has started to grow and develop organs, it no longer is free-floating but needs to be implanted into the uterus, where it is fed by the placenta. It is currently possible to keep (with difficulty, and only for a few days) free-floating embryos alive in enriched culture fluids, but a placental substitute has completely defeated scientific ingenuity. In humans, normal embryos can currently only be kept alive for about the first four or five days after fertilisation; after about six days they start to disintegrate and no human embryo has been cultured for longer than nine days – even though the legal limit is fourteen. It is, however, possible to keep rat embryos alive outside the womb until all the major organs have developed. This is done by keeping them in an organ bath to which nutrients and oxygen are added; diffusion of essential substances into the embryonic tissues is aided by constant agitation of the culture bath. Complete development is not possible and these experiments have largely been done to test drugs and other substances which may be teratogenic, i.e. cause genetic malformations. The implanted embryo needs to get its life-giving nutrients from the placenta which develops and grows with the constantly adapting maternal tissues.

So far, it has not been possible to make an artificial placenta, and this is not surprising because the functions of the placenta are so highly complex. Not only does the placenta provide oxygen and remove carbon dioxide, but it is also responsible for the manufacture of essential proteins, nutrition, control of the blood supply, heat regulation, removal of waste products, manufacture of protecting antibodies, and hormonal regulation of the advancing pregnancy. Any artificial placenta would therefore have to be much more complicated than, for example, our very inexpertly made artificial kidneys, or the crude heart-lung machines which we are able to use for the life-support of humans for a few hours at a time.

I have no doubt that extrauterine foetal life may be possible for humans in the very far future. I do not see this in any way as a threat. I do not believe that there is any likelihood of a Huxleyian conveyor belt, turning out designer babies. In fact, an artificial placenta would literally be a godsend. One of the commonest reasons for babies dying currently is severe prematurity. Premature babies cannot always breathe properly because their lungs are not fully developed, and other organs such as the immature brain and heart cannot cope with the sudden demands made upon them by the early switch between protected intrauterine life and the harsh environment outside the womb. All we can do at present is to put them in a very inadequate environment in a heated, air-filled incubator, where they largely have to fend for themselves. Connecting these babies to some kind of artificial placental system would be a remarkable and important advance in human medicine.

Animal-human hybrids

It has until recently been impossible to create hybrids between different animal species, unless they are very closely related genetically. Sperm from a donkey can fertilise eggs of a horse, producing a mule, because these two animals are very closely related. It is not possible, as far as we know, to cross-breed any monkey with a man, because the genetic relationship is not close enough. The zona pellucida, the surrounding coat of an egg, carries specific receptors which only allow sperm of the same species to penetrate it and cause fertilisation. This outer protective coating might be dissolved in some species to allow cross-fertilisation, but this has never been attempted.

During the recent parliamentary debate on human embryology, some MPs expressed outrage at the hamster egg penetration test (see p. 145). In this test of the fertilising capacity of human sperm, hamster eggs first have the zona artificially dissolved, following which they are exposed to human sperm to see whether or not sperm can penetrate the egg. Successful penetration is regarded as a positive result and evidence of the functional capacity of human sperm. Such 'fertilisation' cannot produce a viable embryo – a 'humster', and therefore the outrage was hardly appropriate. In actual fact, as we have seen, the hamster test is not a particularly useful test anyway, and few laboratories use it.

The Chimaera was a monster in Greek mythology with a lion's head, a goat's body, and a dragon's tail. Somewhat alarmingly, its head continually vomited flame. The Chimaera was the offspring of Echidna, who made rather a habit of this kind of thing, producing the Sphinx, the Hydra and Cerberus, the three-headed dog of Pluto, who guarded the Underworld. It is possible to produce a chimaera (more usually spelt 'chimera') in the laboratory by mixing cells from different embryos very early during development. In practice, scientists have injected embryonic cells from one species of mouse into the embryo of another, and the offspring have inherited the characteristics of both animals. Chimeras have also been produced in rats, rabbits and sheep, and the most famous chimera was the notorious sheep-goat[46] produced by Dr Steen Willadsen in his experiments in Cambridge some years ago. Creating chimeras is not at all a frivolous exercise, because they are a very important model for human disease, and for cell differentiation. Dr Handyside and his colleagues produced chimeras from normal mice mixed with cells from mice with Lesch-Nyhan syndrome, a crippling human condition, which causes severe spasticity.[47] These animals gave very important information about this disease and the way it is expressed genetically. Chimeras have also given us very important information about sexual characteristics. Although the embryonic cells that are mixed may come from two animals of a different sex, chimeras are virtually always of one or other sex, and hermaphrodites are

[46] This rather bedraggled-looking animal with very odd fleece behaved like a goat, but didn't smell like one. It also preferred the company of sheep.

[47] These mice were very interesting, because they clearly could be shown to be expressing the chemical changes caused by the Lesch-Nyhan gene, and passing it on to their offspring. However, the main effect of this gene is to decrease mental acuity; somewhat difficult to test in laboratory mice.

very rare. Oddly most chimeras are male but the reason for this is still not entirely clear. What is more bizarre is that male chimeras, though frequently carrying female chromosomes as well as male chromosomes, are usually fertile males.

Chimeras can actually occur naturally during human development, and are possibly not that uncommon. Cells from twin human embryos can occasionally mix together spontaneously, giving rise to a single person, derived from two separate embryos – yet more evidence that the fertilised human egg is not necessarily a unique individual.

Since the Human Fertilisation and Embryology Act of 1990, it is a criminal offence deliberately to produce a human chimera in Britain, and rightly so. Although animal hybrids of this kind may be of immense experimental importance in researching many aspects of development, it is quite clear that no scientist would tamper with a human in this way.

Embryonic cell lines

The study of cells taken from embryos is of immense importance, and I believe this to be one of the most important areas of research yet to be fully exploited. As yet, virtually no human research has been done, but the study of embryonic cells, grown in culture after removal from an embryo, will undoubtedly give crucial information about how cells differentiate and develop into specialised cell lines. It may be possible to influence this differentiation in due course so that embryonic cells could be produced which are, for an example, pure blood cells or liver cells. Such cells, if growing normally, could be transplanted into humans suffering from fatal diseases such as leukaemia to replace their own diseased cancerous cells. This is an attractive possibility because embryonic cells, being immunologically different from 'adult' cells, may not be subject to rejection by the body. This would avoid the serious problems currently encountered with transplantation of adult organs and cells. In future, it may even be possible to replace damaged nerve or brain cells in this way, for example in the treatment of the common crippling disease, Parkinson's syndrome. The ethical problems with such research and treatments are as yet unresolved, and there is sure to be heated public debate in the future.

Genetic engineering of human embryos

One of the biggest ethical issues concerns genetic engineering in embryos. IVF technology and the possibility of screening embryos for genetic diseases have raised the criticism that doctors, or governments, may try in future to manipulate human embryos so that only embryos with 'desirable' genes are produced. Of course, genetic engineering of humans is rightly banned, but the vision of Nazi Germany is still sufficiently close for decent people to be justifiably concerned that an evil scientist may attempt to misuse a human embryo in this way.

In actual practice, there is very little point in trying to produce humans with desirable characteristics. Fortunately for the human race, attributes like beauty, aggression, tallness, strength, intelligence, persistence, docility and musicality are not the product of single genes, but many different genes working together with influences in the developmental environment. It is extremely unlikely that they could be 'designed' into an embryo. In any case, no fascist dictator would wait the necessary eighteen years after gestation or any genetically engineered embryos to produce a 'master race', or even a decent orchestra. Manipulation of education and environmental factors will always be sadly much more effective in subverting human destiny.

Genetic engineering has also been suggested as a means for combating human disease. The injection of a 'normal' gene into an abnormal embryo is called 'germ-line gene therapy'. Abnormal genes could be replaced by normal genes in defective embryos, so that when they grow up and have children, their offspring would be free of the disease, and free of the status of carrying the abnormal gene. This has therefore been suggested as a way of correcting human gene defects permanently.

There are many serious objections to germ-line gene therapy. First, there is no guarantee that the injection of a given gene would lead to its correct expression in the offspring. Unless a gene is correctly incorporated in the DNA of an embryo, it is highly probable that it will not have the desired beneficial effect. Second, gene injection might dislodge other essential genes from their proper place in the human genome. The effects of this could be catastrophic, because it would cause severe foetal abnormalities. An example of this can be seen from Dr Jon Gordon's work on mice in New York City. He has done important studies producing transgenic animals, animals that have been deliberately treated by gene injection at the early embryonic stage. Transgenic mice are one way that scientists can study effectively the actions of individual genes and the way they are expressed. When I visited his laboratory a few years ago, Dr Gordon showed me some mice in which he had incorporated different human genes,[48] responsible for disease. In one experiment, he had successfully incorporated a gene responsible for certain aspects of bone marrow metabolism – an important experiment, because it has given information about the possible treatment of types of bone marrow cancer. Some of his animals had expressed the gene normally; others showed obvious quite unrelated deformities, such as blindness, absent ears, missing limbs and abnormalities of the tail. Clearly the risks of this happening in a human baby are so serious that it would be a highly irresponsible doctor who would countenance such a possibility. Apart from any humanitarian consideration, it is highly improbable that any doctor would risk this. Not least, he would be liable to huge financial damages for the care of such a child. Third, it is possible that germ-line cell therapy could activate oncogenes, the genes which control cancers. There is serious concern that injecting any gene into an embryo

[48] After leaving, I dreamt that one of these mice escaped and, meeting some friends, produced a weird colony populating the New York sewers.

might activate various cancers and this, of course, makes such therapy out of the question.

In any event, there is another reason why I consider germ-line gene therapy unlikely to be used. Simply, it is unnecessary. Preimplantation diagnosis, described in Chapter 14, would be just as effective in preventing carrier embryos passing on serious genetic disorders, and this has none of these very serious risks.

Finally there is one other very serious moral, theoretical question about genetic engineering. We belong to a species, Homo sapiens. A species is ultimately defined by its genome, its genetic structure. Each species has a unique combination of genes which defines it in evolutionary terms. Were we to produce transgenic humans we would in effect be changing the human species. The consequences of genetic restructuring would be to alter or promote our natural evolution. I think that humans might, in future, have the power to alter our species in some way, thus subverting evolution. This, in the long distant future, is a very serious possibility. Indeed, I think it inevitable that eventually, perhaps many hundreds of years hence, there will be attempts to do this, providing humans survive long enough on the surface of our threatened planet. Hopefully, this will never be done until we can be sure that this would be only for 'human' good. It is an awesome thought to consider that we, who consider ourselves to be made in God's image, may actually change that image in some way. How that would be reconciled with religious and human values is hard to see.

The case against embryo research

I have presented many arguments supporting embryo research. Opposition to it is based partly on moral or religious grounds, and on the fear of a misuse of technology. Some of the other arguments which have been put forward can be summarised as follows:

'HUMAN LIFE BEGINS AT CONCEPTION AND IS SACROSANCT'

This is the most potent of religious arguments. It takes various forms: that the human embryo is a person or that it is 'human' and, as such, is entitled to be protected like any other human.[49] This argument eventually comes down to a matter of belief. Most people find it difficult to accept that the embryo, a mere ball of undifferentiated cells with only limited potential for development, can be equated with a foetus, which has organs and which moves and which at least has a better than even chance of survival in the uterus. It seems to me that our society, by the widespread use of contraceptive methods such as the intrauterine coil (which leads to embryonic destruction) has already decided the status of the human embryo.

'THE HUMAN EMBRYO IS A UNIQUE INDIVIDUAL'

Each embryo has its own unique set of genes, which will give rise to its own unique attributes. However, twins can be formed as late as fourteen days after fertilisation when the 'unique' embryo splits into two. Moreover, human chimeras naturally occur when cells from twin embryos get mixed in the same organism. In any case, 'uniqueness' is not only a property of the embryo; as we have seen, each egg and each sperm are also unique.

[49] Some critics claim also that we are 'creating life' in the test-tube, and thus implying that we are subverting the work of God's creation. But surely we are using the materials given by God? This is a form of *imitatio dei* and, as such, is to be greatly commended in Judaeo-Christian tradition because, made in the image of God, we are here to help His works.

'A TIME LIMIT IS THE START OF A SLIPPERY SLOPE'

A common argument is that if society allows scientists to experiment up to a certain number of days after fertilisation (fourteen days in Britain), scientists will want to extend this period if it becomes expedient or useful to do so. To my mind, this argument is fallacious. The medical profession already has many limits imposed on it concerning what is ethical in research, and these limits are fully and totally accepted. A variation of the argument is that if scientists are allowed to experiment on embryos, they will not stop at a point that is generally acceptable.

'PEOPLE WHO ARE INFERTILE HAVE BROUGHT IT UPON THEMSELVES'

The implication is that research into infertility is not worth while, because infertile people have created their own problem by carelessness or promiscuous behaviour. The argument runs along the lines of 'Why get into grey moral areas for the sake of people who are not worthy?' This remarkably callous and unfair argument was presented by more than one politician during debates on embryo research.

'ANY RESEARCH THAT IS NEEDED CAN BE DONE USING ANIMALS'

Animal research is most important in understanding human reproduction; indeed, it is vital that animal research continue. One of the most important research centres has been the London Zoo, which is sadly now threatened with closure but which has conducted very important work in this field. Unfortunately, study of animal embryos is not a complete substitute for human research. Animals do not suffer the same genetic diseases as humans, they have different genes and chromosomes, rarely have miscarriages, virtually never suffer ectopic pregnancy, and are, in general, far more fertile.

The campaign against embryo research

Many of these arguments came to a head before the recent parliamentary legislation (1991) which finally permitted human embryo research under strict controls. There was growing awareness in the early 1980s that IVF technology involved the generation of surplus embryos. It was also realised that genetic manipulation, cloning, animal hybrids and human embryo storage were matters of public concern.

The Warnock Committee was established by the British government to look into these and related areas. Having taken copious evidence over two years, the committee concluded that embryo research was of substantial benefit. It recommended that embryo research should be permitted up to fourteen days after fertilisation, when the first signs of embryonic differentiation and organ growth occur and when implantation is largely completed. Fourteen days, incidentally, is also when a woman might perceive that she is pregnant as that is the time when she would miss her period. The committee made a number of recommendations, in particular that a government licensing authority be set up to regulate matters relating to IVF, donor insemination, fertility treatments and embryo research.

The government was slow to react. Although debates on the report followed in both Houses of Parliament (and many MPs were concerned about embryo research), no government bill was introduced. The government felt it had more pressing business. A powerful lobby, led mainly by the two organisations Life and the Society for the Protection of the Unborn Child, called for a ban on embryo research. They sought a Member of Parliament who would take up the issue, and were fortunate when that great champion of causes, Mr Enoch Powell, won the Private Member's Ballot to introduce a bill at the end of 1984.

Mr Powell's Unborn Children (Protection) Bill received its second reading on 15 February 1985. In his opening speech on that day, Mr Powell emphasised his feeling of 'revulsion and repugnance' at the destruction of embryos 'for the purpose of the acquisition of knowledge'. Some listeners found it odd that Mr Powell did not appear to sense the same 'revulsion' at embryos being destroyed (daily, in their thousands) by that popular method of contraception the IUD (coil). Was it then the 'acquisition of knowledge' that caused Mr Powell so much personal distress? The ensuing debate was extremely revealing. Most MPs opposed to embryo research displayed remarkable ignorance about what was involved. In spite of numerous invitations from researchers, very few of them, including Mr Powell, had bothered to visit a department where embryo research was being conducted.

Mr Powell's bill had many glaring deficiences. It required, for example, that all women having IVF treatment would require prior permission in writing from the Secretary of State. This infringement of personal liberty, completely unparalleled in any other medical treatment, was accepted without question by his supporters in the House of Commons, who mustered an astonishing majority of 172 votes at the second reading. This was particularly remarkable as Mr Powell's bill aimed to ban all research on embryos, except *where researched embryos were to be transferred back to the womb*. The appalling consequences of this – that women might deliver children which had been made abnormal by research – were pointed out to him, but he remained intransigent on this issue, as on virtually every other.

Although Enoch Powell's bill failed to get a third reading, it is remarkable that there were four more attempts to revive it. The last, in February 1989, was an identically worded bill introduced in the House of Lords by the Duke of Norfolk. The Duke, who is the lay leader of the Catholic Church in Britain, and a fine and humanitarian man, at least took great trouble to brief himself properly by visiting research units before his bill. Nevertheless he seemed to ignore the many glaring anomalies in Mr Powell's bill; many people believe he was under pressure from the Roman Catholic Church to introduce such legislation.

Perhaps his heart was not fully in it because, when he realised that his opponents were to introduce numerous amendments at the committee stages, he withdrew his bill (April 1989).

Not all parliamentary activity was negative. An all-party parliamentary group called PROGRESS was set up after Mr Powell's bill foundered. It has been very influential in helping politicians understand why embryo research is essential. Many organisations involved with health care or handicap have joined PROGRESS, which still has important work to do if reproductive research is to be protected. PROGRESS needs membership; should you be interested in supporting its activities, please write to the address on p. 349.

Government legislation on reproductive technology

In November 1987 the government produced a White Paper on reproductive technology. It proposed setting up a licensing authority to regulate in vitro fertilisation, with a free vote on the question of embryo research. Although the White Paper was extensively debated, no government bill was immediately forthcoming. Doctors and scientists were left to regulate themselves. In 1985 the Royal College of Obstetricians and Gynaecologists, together with the Medical Research Council, founded the Voluntary Licensing Authority (VLA). This was an interim measure until government legislation was passed. In fact, the VLA continued to police IVF in the absence of government control, and did so very effectively. There was never a single case of unethical or dangerous research, and all clinics voluntarily submitted to inspection, agreeing to the VLA guidelines. None the less, continued pressure on parliament eventually made legislation inevitable.

In 1990, after intense campaigning by many right-to-life groups, a parliamentary struggle commenced. The government decided on a free vote, allowing MPs to vote according to their conscience rather than along party lines. Remarkable things happened and emotions were extraordinarily high. The debate was passionate, but on the whole well informed and sensitive. It was completely unclear how the vote would eventually go, but finally, at 11.00 p.m. on 23 April 1990, the debating chamber filled dramatically and parliament voted overwhelmingly by 173 votes in favour of allowing embryo research. It is fair to say that the House of Commons was in uproar with the vote; I saw hardened Members of the Commons embracing each other with tears running down their cheeks when they realised that a major victory for common sense and humanity had been won.

Of course issues involving human reproduction raise strong feelings. Nobody doubts the sincerity of those who believe that the human embryo is a person entitled to full protection. However, that clearly is a minority view: over the last five years in Britain there have been several national opinion polls and one medical research study, all of which indicate that the majority of British people feels that embryo research is right, particularly if used to combat genetic disease. When parliament did finally vote on the issue, it recognised that we live in a pluralistic society. In such a society, the individual families affected by these catastrophic diseases should be allowed to have the final say in whether or not their own fertilised eggs may be used to alleviate their suffering. Parliament also struck an important blow for infertile couples, raising the profile of the suffering caused by reproductive diseases, and emphasised its trust in the scientists and doctors doing ethical research.

The Human Fertilisation and Embryology Authority (HFEA)

The Human Fertilisation and Embryology Authority Act (November 1990), which followed the parliamentary debate, allowed embryo research for the first fourteen days after fertilisation. The Human Fertilisation and Embryology Authority (HFEA) was set up, and this body was empowered to inspect and regulate all clinics undertaking IVF treatments or donor insemination, and all laboratories doing embryo research.

In addition to regulating research, the main functions of the HFEA include the licensing of clinics storing eggs, sperm and embryos, to publish details of the services that IVF clinics provide, to give advice and information to clinics where appropriate, to publish a code of practice (guidelines) for clinics, and to provide advice and information to donors of sperm or eggs. The authority currently has twenty-one members, of whom six are medically qualified. The remainder are scientists or lay members. So far it has licensed 106 centres, amongst which sixty-eight are licensed for IVF, and seventeen for research.

FUNDING THE HFEA

The HFEA is quite a costly body to run. It has over 100 centres to visit, inspect and license each year, it has to collect and collate a good deal of data from clinics and has developed a considerable committee infrastructure, which advises it on various matters such as ethical issues. It also undoubtedly generates a mound of paperwork, which at times seems rather excessive to hard-pressed infertility clinics. After the first year in action the HFEA has published an annual report, a very glossy booklet in which coloured photographs of various members of the HFEA are prominently displayed. This does not seem to be a particularly good way of spending money, and has raised the anger of many doctors and patients.

Many professionals, myself included, are very concerned that although the HFEA is a body set up by the government to regulate on its behalf, its activities are only partly funded by Whitehall. The rest of the money has to be raised by clinics carrying out treatment, who pay a licence fee – one for IVF and storage of eggs or sperm, and one for each research project undertaken. Each IVF treatment cycle is also subject to a treatment fee, currently £30, and there is no guarantee that this fee will not be increased.

Most people involved with IVF treatment feel that licence fees are unjust. It is certainly unprecedented. There is no other medical treatment which is subject to comparable fees, and I know of no situation where patients are put in the position of paying for the regulation of their own treatment. This is denying a responsibility which is properly that of central government. This system has caused hardship in my own clinic and has prevented us from offering more NHS treatments than we do. What is shocking is that infertility treatment is already severely underfunded in this country and this extra impost is perceived as yet another example of the plight of infertile people being slighted. Although hotly denied by many politicians and officials, IVF fees are seen by ordinary patients as a taxation on infertility.

REGULATING RESEARCH

The research which has been conducted has been effectively regulated by the HFEA and is of real human value. Projects currently licensed cover:

1. Improving infertility treatments:
    a. improving the environmental conditions for culturing embryos;
    b. estimation of the energy requirements of human embryos;
    c. methods for improving fertilisation of eggs;
    d. attempts to improve implantation of human embryos.
2. Improving means of storage of eggs, sperm and embryos.
3. Better diagnosis and treatment of genetic disorders:
    a. preimplantation research; how chromosomal disorders occur;
    b. gene expression in human embryos.
4. Development of contraceptive vaccines.

All these projects are conducted within the fourteen-day

limit laid down by parliament, and all have important applications for improving various medical treatments. Their regulation is relatively easy, as it is virtually impossible for a centre to do unauthorised research without being caught. In any case, scientists only benefit from research when they publish their results. Publication is only possible with ethical and HFEA approval, as no scientific journal will accept material without such approval. So far, the projects on improving culture conditions and genetic diagnosis have already been of significant benefit, and healthy children have been born in consequence of this research.

REGULATING CLINICAL PRACTICE

The HFEA has very firmly set out to regulate clinical practice. It tries to influence how IVF treatments are done by formulating a code of practice to which centres are expected to adhere. This is controversial and, in my view, it is virtually impossible effectively (or sensibly) to control how doctors do their work, what patients they accept for treatment, how much they charge for their services, or what advice they give to patients. The HFEA also lays great stress on the provision of counselling services for patients, but this is a major problem, because very few trained infertility counsellors are available. Moreover, the NHS has consistently refused to pay for counselling, and the private clinics are reluctant to spend the sums of money required to employ adequate, independent counsellors. The effectiveness of the HFEA in these important areas, which at present seems quite limited, remains to be seen.

PUBLICATION OF RESULTS

A prospective patient should undoubtedly receive accurate, unbiased information about a given clinic's results before undergoing treatment. The HFEA collects data on all centres and publishes statistics, together with the range of success:

344 PROBLEMS DURING EARLY PREGNANCY

CLINIC SIZE* (number of clinics in brackets)	PATIENTS	IVF CYCLES	PREGNANCIES RANGE	BIRTHS RANGE
Large (8)	5,218	6,165	2.7%–29.3%	2.1%–22.9%
Medium (21)	3,814	4,365	3.5%–28.6%	2.3%–23.3%
Small (35)	932	1,053	0.0%–45.0%	0.0%–33.3%
TOTAL:	9,964	11,583	2,004 (17.3%)	1,443 (12.5%)

* Table taken from the HFEA Annual Report, 1992. Compare this table with that on p. 226

Although one or two small clinics (treating fewer than 100 cycles annually) have a very high success rate – this is almost certainly a statistical quirk, due to very small numbers treated – in general, the eight largest clinics (over 400 cycles annually) are the most successful. Although these are most successful, one of the most alarming statistics is that, amongst the eight 'leading' clinics, there is a staggering tenfold difference in success rate. Incidentally, most of these 'leading clinics' are private, with patients paying substantial fees for their services. An unsuspecting couple could easily find themselves paying for treatment in a clinic with only a 2.1 per cent success rate and not know any better. This clearly shows the limitations of the HFEA figures. The greatest controversy concerns the possibility of having a 'league table' but unless the HFEA is prepared to publish such a 'league table' of success rates, patients are bound to remain ignorant of their true expectations.

This is a knotty problem which the HFEA has so far failed to grasp. It is difficult to accept that the HFEA is doing an effective job until it is prepared to offer better guidance to IVF patients.

Prospects for the future

Throughout this book I have highlighted the problems in reproductive medicine, and where I think necessary I have been critical of much medical practice. It must be clear that the NHS often provides a very inadequate service, sometimes scandalously poor. Far too often patients with reproductive problems are relegated to the most junior, inexperienced doctor on the team, patients see a different doctor at each visit, there are long waiting lists and, most reprehensible, too many NHS consultants show scant appreciation of the importance of infertility medicine and the sad plight of couples who need it.

People often believe that they will do much better by 'going private'. Of course there are some good private clinics, but in my view much of the private sector falls very far short of ideal. Indeed, many private clinics offer worse treatment than that available under the NHS. Some private treatment exploits the desperation of infertile couples, some private clinics are staffed by individuals who are poorly trained or ignorant, and there are far too many private IVF clinics that can only offer IVF. A patient going to such a clinic may well end up having IVF when there may be a far simpler, cheaper treatment which is 'inconvenient' in a commercial setting. At the present time, there are private clinics eagerly falling over themselves to attract customers, and this is an unhealthy situation.[50]

Fortunately, there is real hope for the future of reproductive medicine. This is surely in the public sector, where it can be properly regulated, and where it will undoubtedly improve. The public sector has made nearly all the major advances in research,[51] and there is growing enthusiasm for good academic

[50] I admit to having been heavily criticised by many 'colleagues' for these views on private practice, who take grave exception to them. At times my life has been made miserable because I have dared to step out of line. Oddly, whilst I have come under the heaviest fire for expressing unpopular views on private clinics, I never once have been condemned for publicly expressing quite similar views about the NHS. Readers may draw their own conclusions.

[51] This is denied by private clinics which claim to have made important

work in this field in university hospitals. The Royal College of Obstetricians and Gynaecologists has set up a proper training programme in reproduction, and professional organisations such as the British Fertility Society increasingly attract young specialists in training, where they can present their research work and learn from others. The HFEA has the power, and the will, to help improve patient management and the Medical Research Council is setting aside a major proportion of its budget for high quality research. Most important, general practitioners – the family doctors – are beginning to understand the importance of this field and are increasingly offering better advice to patients. Above all, patients themselves are becoming more educated and more critical. Patient-orientated organisations such as ISSUE and CHILD are increasingly effective bodies and there will be growing pressure on the Department of Health and NHS hospitals to ensure substantial improvements. The sad thing is that all this takes time, and speed is needed if today's patients are going to benefit by tomorrow's advances.

---

innovative advances, but the scientific literature suggests otherwise. The evidence is quite clear: for example, 90 per cent of IVF treatments are made in the private sector, but according to the HFEA Annual Report, of the thirty-three licensed research projects, all but three are being conducted on university or NHS premises.

SUGGESTED READING

Houghton, Diane and Peter, *Coping with Childlessness*, George Allen & Unwin, London, 1984. A fine book describing the feelings and experience of infertility; admirably critical and very honest.

Jones, Maggie, *Everything You Need to Know about Adoption*, Sheldon Press, London, 1987. A useful account of all aspects of adoption, practical and business-like.

Leese, Henry, *Human Reproduction and* In Vitro *Fertilisation*, Macmillan Education, London, 1988. This is a clear and detailed account written by one of the most respected and innovative scientists in the field. Excellent background for those who want readable, in-depth information on IVF.

Pfeffer, Naomi, and Anne Woolett, *The Experience of Infertility*, Virago Press, London, 1983. Still my favourite book on the feelings that people, especially women, have about infertility. The authors show great concern and sensitivity. A feminist book with great comfort to people with intractable infertility. The medical information in it is not always entirely accurate.

Pizer, Hank, and Christine O'Brien Palinski, *Coping with a Miscarriage*, Jill Norman, London, 1980. This deals with the medical and emotional aspects of miscarriage; it contains much useful information, though some is now a little out of date.

Rothman, Barbara Katz, *The Tentative Pregnancy: Prenatal diagnosis and the future of motherhood*, Pandora Press, London, 1988. This is a particularly sensitive account of the problems involved in antenatal genetic screening and the decision-making process.

Snowden, Robert, *The Gift of a Child*, George Allen & Unwin, London, 1984. This is still the most useful book for couples contemplating the decisions involved in donor insemination.

USEFUL ADDRESSES

United Kingdom

BRITISH AGENCIES FOR ADOPTION AND FOSTERING
11 SOUTHWARK STREET, LONDON SE1 1RQ
(071-407 8800)

Promotes good practice in adoption and publishes a useful guide.

CHILD
PO BOX 154, HOUNSLOW TW5 OEZ
(081-571 4367)

CHILD is a charitable organisation designed to promote the welfare of infertile couples, and to offer them support. It publishes a regular newsletter, has a telephone hotline for members, and has regional and national meetings. Most of its members are couples who have been treated for infertility.

ENDOMETRIOSIS ASSOCIATION
65 HOLMDENE AVENUE, HERNE HILL, LONDON SE24 9LD
(071-737 4764)

Self-help group with a useful newsletter and various nationwide contact groups for sufferers with this disease.

FAMILY PLANNING ASSOCIATION (FPA)
27–35 MORTIMER STREET, LONDON W1N 7RJ
(071-631 0555)

THE HUMAN FERTILISATION AND EMBRYOLOGY AUTHORITY
PAXTON HOUSE, 30 ARTILLERY LANE, LONDON E1 7LS
(071-377 5077)

HFEA is the government regulatory body which licenses clinics and is responsible for overseeing that proper standards are maintained in IVF clinics, and that treatment with donor eggs, sperm and embryos is done correctly.

ISSUE
(formerly the National Association for the Childless)
ST GEORGE'S RECTORY, TOWER STREET, BIRMINGHAM B19 3UY
(021-359 4887)

ISSUE is similar in its aims to CHILD. It publishes an increasingly professional journal, has information sheets for potential patients, and, like CHILD, hotline support, an excellent regional network, and a list of clinics.

MISCARRIAGE ASSOCIATION
18 STONEYBROOK CLOSE, WEST BRETTON, WAKEFIELD WF4 4TP
(092-484515)

Support group and help for women who have had miscarriages. Newsletter and information pamphlets available.

MULTIPLE BIRTHS ASSOCIATION
INSTITUTE OF OBSTETRICS AND GYNAECOLOGY, QUEEN
CHARLOTTE'S MATERNITY HOSPITAL, GOLDHAWK ROAD, LONDON W6
(081-748 4666)

Runs support and advice for families with multiple births, and acts as an extremely effective pressure group.

PROGRESS
27–35 MORTIMER STREET, LONDON WC1
(071-436 4528)

PROGRESS has a committee, part lay, part politician and partly scientific. It is politically orientated and promotes the cause of reproductive research issues in Britain and, increasingly, in Europe. It has been an extremely effective lobby group and has looked after rights of patients extremely effectively, often without huge publicity.

ROYAL COLLEGE OF OBSTETRICIANS AND GYNAECOLOGISTS
27 SUSSEX PLACE, REGENT'S PARK, LONDON NW1 4RG
(071-262 5425)

The Royal College is the professional body to which all qualified gynaecologists in Britain belong. It sets standards for their training, and has a growing and important interest in human reproduction which it increasingly sees as a major sub-speciality.

New Zealand

AUCKLAND INFERTILITY SOCIETY INC.
PO BOX 68428 AUCKLAND

AUCKLAND WOMEN'S HEALTH COLLECTIVE
THE WOMEN'S CENTRE, 63 PONSONBY ROAD, AUCKLAND
Tel: 0-9-3764506

CHRISTCHURCH INFERTILITY SOCIETY INC.
PO BOX 29188 CHRISTCHURCH

FAMILY PLANNING ASSOCIATION
REGIONAL OFFICE, MARGARET SPARROW CENTRE, 2ND FLOOR,
45 TONY STREET, PO BOX 9574, WELLINGTON
Tel: 0-4-3849744

FAMILY PLANNING ASSOCIATION
REGIONAL OFFICE, 30 PONSONBY ROAD, PO BOX 68–245, NEWTON,
AUCKLAND
Tel: 0–9–3600360

FAMILY PLANNING ASSOCIATION
REGIONAL OFFICE, ARTS CENTRE, 301 MONTREAL STREET,
PO BOX 2137, CHRISTCHURCH
Tel: 0–3–3790514

FAMILY PLANNING ASSOCIATION
REGIONAL OFFICE, 95 HANOVER STREET, PO BOX 5298, DUNEDIN
Tel: 0–3–4775850

FERTILITY ACTION
2ND FLOOR, 27 GILLIES AVENUE, NEWMARKET, PO BOX 4569,
AUCKLAND 1
Tel: 0–9–5205295

THE HEALTH ALTERNATIVE FOR WOMEN (THAW)
CRANMER CENTRE, CNR MONTREAL AND ARMAGH STREETS,
PO BOX 884, CHRISTCHURCH
Tel: 0–3–3796970

OTAGO/SOUTHLAND INFERTILITY SOCIETY INC.
PO BOX 6286, DUNEDIN NORTH

WELLINGTON INFERTILITY SOCIETY INC.
PO BOX 31279 LOWER HUTT

INDEX